Official Journal of the American Society of Pediatric Neurosurgery (ASPN)

Pediatric Neurosurgery

Founded 1985 by E.B. Hendrick and D.H. Reigel
(formerly 'Pediatric Neuroscience')

KARGER

Printed in Switzerland
on acid-free paper by
Thür AG Offsetdruck, Pratteln

Appears bimonthly:
1 volume per year (6 issues)

Instructions to Authors

Pediatric Neurosurgery

Submission: Only original papers written in English are considered and should be sent to:

Dr. Donald H. Reigel, MD
Managing Editor
Pediatric Neurosurgery
Allegheny General Hospital
East Wing, Suite 212
320 E. North Avenue
Pittsburgh, PA 15212 (USA)

Manuscripts should be submitted in triplicate (with three sets of illustrations of which one is an original), typewritten double-spaced on one side of the paper, with a wide margin.

Conditions: All manuscripts are subject to editorial review. Manuscripts are received with the explicit understanding that they are not under simultaneous consideration by any other publication. Submission of an article for publication implies the transfer of the copyright from the author to the publisher upon acceptance. Accepted papers become the permanent property of 'Pediatric Neurosurgery' and may not be reproduced by any means, in whole or in part, without the written consent of the publisher. It is the author's responsibility to obtain permission to reproduce illustrations, tables, etc. from other publications.

Arrangement:
Title page: The first page of each paper should indicate the title (main title underlined), the authors' names, and the institute where the work was conducted. A translation of the full title into English and a short title for use as running head as well as the full address of the author to whom correspondence should be sent are also required.
Full address: The exact postal address complete with postal code must be given at the bottom of the title page. Please also supply Phone and Fax numbers.
Key words: For indexing purposes, a list of 3 - 10 key words in English is essential.
Abstract: Each paper needs an abstract of up to 10 lines.
Small type: Paragraphs which can or must be set in smaller type (case histories, test methods, etc.) should be indicated with a 'p' (petit) in the margin on the left-hand side.
Footnotes: Avoid footnotes. When essential, they are numbered consecutively and typed at the foot of the appropriate page.
Tables and illustrations: Tables and illustrations (both numbered in Arabic numerals) should be prepared on separate sheets. Tables require a heading and figures a legend, also prepared on a separate sheet. For the reproduction of illustrations, only good drawings and original photographs can be accepted; negatives or photocopies cannot be used. When possible, group several illustrations on one block for reproduction (max. size 181 × 223 mm) or provide crop marks. On the back of each illustration, indicate its number, the author's name, and 'top'. Color illustrations are reproduced at the author's expense.
References: In the text identify references by Arabic numerals [in square brackets]. Material submitted for publication but not yet accepted should be noted as 'unpublished data' and not be included in the reference list. The list of references should include only those publications which are cited in the text. Do not alphabetize; number references in the order in which they are first mentioned in the text. The surnames of the authors followed by initials should be given. There should be no punctuation other than a comma to separate the authors. Cite all authors, 'et al' is not sufficient. Abbreviate journal names according to the Index Medicus system. (Also see International Committee of Medical Journal Editors: Uniform requirements for manuscripts submitted to biomedical journals. Br Med J 1988;296:401–405.)
Examples
(a) Papers published in periodicals: Kauffman HF, van der Heide S, Beaumont F, Blok H, de Vries K: Class-specific antibody determination against *Aspergillus fumigatus* by means of the enzyme-linked immunosorbent assay. III. Comparative study: IgG, IgA, IgM ELISA titers, precipitating antibodies and IgE binding after fractionation of the antigen. Int Arch Allergy Appl Immunol 1986;80:300–306.
(b) Monographs: Matthews DE, Farewell VT: Using and Understanding Medical Statistics. Basel, Karger, 1985.
(c) Edited books: Hardy WD Jr, Essex M: FeLV-induced feline acquired immune deficiency syndrome: A model for human AIDS; in Klein E (ed): Acquired Immunodeficiency Syndrome. Prog Allergy. Basel, Karger, 1986, vol 37, pp 353–376.
Further details: Authors may consult our leaflet 'Rules for the Preparation of Manuscripts', available on request from the Publisher, S. Karger AG, P.O. Box, CH - 4009 Basel (Switzerland).

Galley proofs: Unless indicated otherwise, galley proofs are sent to the first-named author and should be returned with the least possible delay. Alterations made in galley proofs, other than the correction of printer's errors, are charged to the author. No page proofs are supplied.

Reprints: Order forms and a price list are sent with the galley proofs. Orders submitted after the issue is printed are subject to considerably higher prices. Allow five weeks from date of publication for delivery of reprints.

KARGER

General Information

Pediatric Neurosurgery

Publication data: 'Pediatric Neurosurgery' is published 6 times annually. Volume 18 with 6 issues appears in 1992.
Subscription rates: Subscriptions run for a full calendar year. Prices are given per volume, surface postage included.

Personal subscription:	SFr. 213.–,	US$ 142.00.
(Must be in the name of, billed to, and paid by an individual. Order must be marked 'personal subscription'.)		
Residents:	SFr. 127.80,	US$ 80.20.
Institutional subscription:		
(Regular rate.)	SFr. 426.–,	US$ 284.00.
Airmail postage:	SFr. 35.–,	US$ 30.00.
(Extra per volume.)		
Microform subscription:	SFr. 213.–,	US$ 142.00.
(Available exclusively to subscribers of the paper edition.)		

Single issues and back volumes: Information on availability and prices can be obtained through the Publisher.
Advertising: Correspondence and rate requests should be addressed to the Publisher.

Subscription orders: Orders can be placed at agencies, bookstores, directly with the Publisher S. Karger AG, P.O. Box, CH-4009 Basel (Switzerland) or with any of the following distributors:
Deutschland:
S. Karger GmbH, Lörracher Strasse 16A
Postfach, D-W-7800 Freiburg
France: Librairie Luginbühl
36, bd de Latour-Maubourg, F-75007 Paris
Great Britain, Ireland:
S. Karger Publishers, 11 Ravenscroft Road
Beckenham, Kent BR3 4TP
USA: S. Karger Publishers, Inc.
26 West Avon Road, P.O. Box 529
Farmington, CT 06085
India, Bangladesh, Sri Lanka:
S. Karger India Subscription Agency
B-5/132 Safdarjung Enclave
New Delhi-110029
Japan: Katakura Libri, Inc.
36-9 Hongo 3-chome, Bunkyo-ku, Tokyo 113
Change of address: Both old and new address should be stated and sent to the subscription source.

Bibliographic indices: This journal is regularly listed in bibliographic services, including *Current Contents®*.
Book Reviews: Books are accepted for review by special agreement.

KARGER

Horizons of Pediatric Neuroimaging

Guest Editor
Robert A. Zimmerman, Philadelphia, Pa., USA

66 figures, 2 color plates and 4 tables, 1992

KARGER

S. Karger
Medical and Scientific Publishers
Basel · Freiburg · Paris · London
New York · New Delhi · Bangkok
Singapore · Tokyo · Sydney

Drug Dosage
The authors and the publisher have exerted every effort to ensure that drug selection and dosage set forth in this text are in accord with current recommendations and practice at the time of publication. However, in view of ongoing research, changes in government regulations, and the constant flow of information relating to drug therapy and drug reactions, the reader is urged to check the package insert for each drug for any change in indications and dosage and for added warnings and precautions. This is particularly important when the recommended agent is a new and/or infrequently employed drug.

P.O. Box, CH-4009 Basel (Switzerland)
Printed in Switzerland on acid-free paper by
Thür AG Offsetdruck, Pratteln
ISBN 3-8055-5694-2

Contents

Neuroimaging in Pediatric Neurosurgery

Robert A. Zimmerman

The Children's Hospital of Philadelphia, Pa., USA

This special issue of *Pediatric Neurosurgery* is devoted to recent contributions of pediatric neuroradiology to pediatric neurosurgery. Neuroimaging has moved at a rapid pace during the decade of the 80s. We have all made the leap forward from CT to MR imaging. Ultrasound has also shown a similar steady progress. In this issue, the contributors have reviewed several highlights that these changes in neurodiagnosis have brought to neurosurgery. Dr. Richard Smith has reviewed intracranial infection, emphasizing the contributions of magnetic resonance imaging. Dr. James Barkovich has put into perspective the current evaluation of hydrocephalus by neuroimaging. Dr. Otsubo and Dr. Chuang et al. have given us an insight into the utility of different imaging modalities in epileptic patients who are surgical candidates. I have had the opportunity of reviewing the use of MR in diagnosis of pediatric posterior fossa tumors, while Dr. Diane Babcock and associates have put intraoperative ultrasound into perspective. There is little question that we accept each new step forward and hold back our amazement that it will not end. In future issues of *Pediatric Neurosurgery,* we will bring you the future improvements.

Pediatr Neurosurg 1992;18:58–64

Robert A. Zimmerman
Larissa T. Bilaniuk
Susan Rebsamen

Department of Radiology, The Children's Hospital of Philadelphia, Pa., USA

Magnetic Resonance Imaging of Pediatric Posterior Fossa Tumors

Key Words
MRI, brain tumors
Brain tumors, pediatric
Brainstem tumors
Cerebellar tumors
Primitive neuroectodermal tumors
Pilocytic astrocytomas
Ependymomas

Abstract
MR detected abnormality in all 115 pediatric patients who subsequently had pathologically proven posterior fossa tumors. In 114, the initial magnetic resonance (MR) diagnosis was that of brain tumor. In 1, with less than 1-cm^2 area of gadolinium enhancement, the significance of the initial finding was uncertain. Common posterior fossa tumor subgroups (brainstem gliomas, cerebellar astrocytomas, primitive neuroectodermal tumors, and ependymomas) have relatively consistent presentations on imaging studies. However, less common tumors mimic the MR appearance of more common ones, while common tumors may also have atypical appearances.

Introduction

The greater sensitivity of magnetic resonance (MR) over computed tomography (CT) in the detection of posterior fossa tumors in the pediatric patient has been demonstrated over the past 8 years [1, 2]. However, the question that persists is how often do the MR findings correlate to the tumor types when classified pathologically. It is recognized with MR that localization of the mass to either the cerebellum, brainstem, fourth ventricle, cerebellopontine angle or investing meninges and calvarial vault is the first step in arriving at a differential diagnosis [1, 2]. The sites to which the tumor mass extends, its signal characteristics on various pulse sequences, and its enhancement characteristics following gadolinium injection, are also used to further characterize the tumor type [3]. Clinical information, such as the type of clinical signs and symptoms and their rate of progression, provides further information useful in narrowing the imaging differential diagnosis [3]. This paper focuses on the reliability and pitfalls found in imaging characteristics in a series of 115 histologically proven tumors taken from a total of 141 MR newly diagnosed pediatric posterior fossa tumors.

Methods and Materials

A retrospective review was carried out of the MR findings in all newly diagnosed pediatric posterior fossa tumors seen at The Children's Hospital of Philadelphia from January 1987 through October 1991 (58 months). One hundred and forty-one patients with tumors were studied, for which pathology was obtained in 115 (82%). Twenty-six tumors without pathologic confirmation consisted of 23 brainstem masses thought to represent gliomas, and 3 instances of bilateral acoustic neuromas associated with type II neurofibromatosis. Sex distribution for the 141 patients was 85 males and 56 females. Patients ranged in age from birth to age 18.

All patients were studied in a 1.5-Tesla MR unit. All studies were performed with similar spin echo pulse sequences, which included a T1-weighted image (T1WI) (TR = 600 ms; TE = 15–20 ms), a proton density-weighted image (PDWI) and T2-weighted image (T2WI) (TR = 3,000 ms; TE = 30 and 80–90 ms) and beginning in October 1988, enhancement with gadolinium DTPA (Magnevist, Berlex Laboratories, Cedar Knolls, N.J; 0.1 mmol/kg) utilizing flow compensation and a TR of 600 ms and a TE of 22–30 ms. Postgadolinium images were obtained in at least two of three cardinal planes (axial, coronal, sagittal). All slices were 5 mm thick, with an interslice gap of no more than 1–2 mm, a matrix size of 192 × 256 to 256 × 256, and were performed with one acquisition.

Robert A. Zimmerman, MD
Department of Radiology
Children's Hospital of Philadelphia
34th Street and Civic Center Boulevard
Philadelphia, PA 19104–4038 (USA)

1016–2291/92/0182–0058
$2.75/0

Results

Anatomic distribution of tumors is given in table 1. Pathology of the tumors is given in table 2. The signal intensity, cystic versus solid, and enhancement characteristics for each type of pathologically proven tumor are given in tables 3 and 4.

Discussion

In this series of pediatric posterior fossa tumors the most common tumor location was the cerebellum (78/115 = 67.8%) (table 1) and the most common tumor pathology was primitive neuroectodermal tumor (PNET) (42/115 tumors = 36.5%; 40/78 cerebellar tumors = 51.3%) (table 2). The PNET arose outside the cerebellum in two instances, both within the brainstem (2/42 PNET = 4.8%) (table 2). Within the brainstem the PNET was an unusual tumor (2/25 histologically proven tumors = 8%) (2/48 total brainstem tumors = 4.17%) (tables 1, 2). On T1WI the PNET was uniformly hypointense to grey matter (42/42 = 100%), a finding that was also present in most other tumors (70/73 = 95.9%) and therefore was not useful in their differential diagnosis (table 3). However, the PNET was most often isointense to cortex on T2WI (40/42 = 95.2%) (fig. 1a), a signal intensity finding that was seen in only two other tumors (1 lymphoma, 1 gliofibroma) (table 4). Both of these tumors could be mistaken for the PNET on the T1WI, T2WI and the gadolinium-enhanced T1WI. This finding on the T2WI in the PNET, lymphoma and gliofibroma is in contrast to the finding of hyperintensity on T2WI in the majority of other tumors (66/72 = 91.7%) (table 3) (fig. 2a).

All but two of the PNETs enhanced with contrast (20/22 = 90.9%) (fig. 1b) as did most other tumors (54/73 = 74%) (table 3; fig. 2b). Intrinsic brainstem gliomas (15/21 = 71.4%) showed the highest percentage of nonenhancement within any group of tumors (fig. 3b). This was most common for pontine tumors that were subsequently diagnosed as malignant (11/13 = 84.6%) at or prior to death (tables 2, 3). The PNET was found to be a noncystic tumor in 42/42 = 100%, a finding common to most other

Table 1. Anatomic site of tumors

Site	All tumors	Tumors with pathologic verification
Brainstem	48	25
Cerebellum	78	78
4th ventricle	11	11
Cerebellopontine angle	3	0
Posterior fossa (specific site of origin not definable)	1	1
Total	141	115

Table 2. Histologic type of tumor and frequency according to location

Pathology	Location				
	brain-stem	cere-bellum	4th ventricle	specific site of origin not definable	total
PNET	2	40			42
Pilocytic astrocytoma		23			23
Malignant glioma	13	4			17
Fibrillary astrocytoma	5	3			8
Astrocytoma	3	4			7
Mixed astrocytoma		1			1
Ganglioglioma		1			1
Gliofibroma			1		1
Medulloepithelioma	1	1			2
Hemangioblastoma	1				1
Lymphoma		1			1
Malignant teratoma				1	1
Ependymoma			10		10
Total	25	78	11	1	115

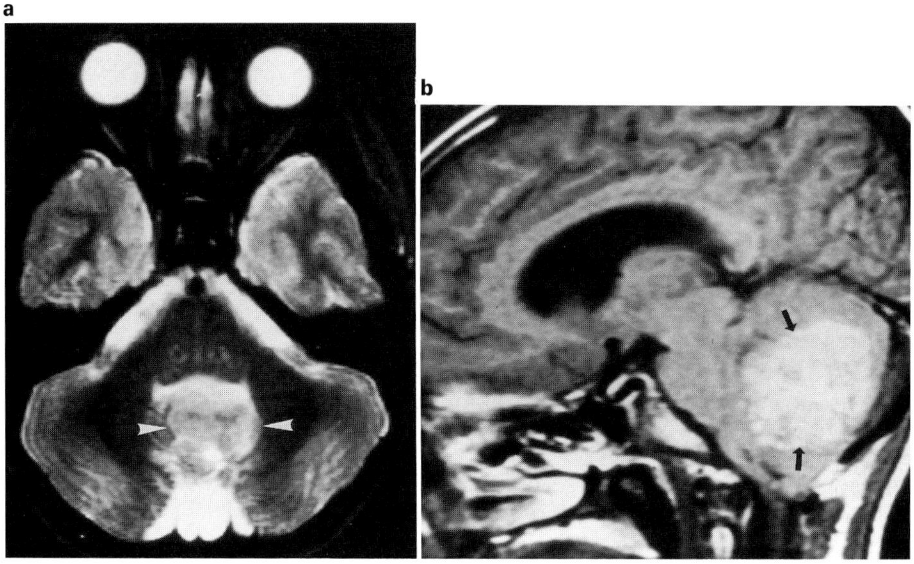

Fig. 1. PNET. **a** Axial T2WI of a 7-year-old male shows a mass lesion of the vermis that is isointense to cortex (arrowheads). **b** Sagittal T1WI postgadolinium injection of a 10-year-old male shows contrast enhancement of a vermian mass (arrows).

Table 3. MR characteristics of specific histologic types of tumors

	Hypointense on T1[a]	Hyperintense on T2WI[a]	Enhancement on T1[a]	Contains cystic component
PNET	42/42	0/42	20/22	0
Pilocytic astrocytoma	23/23	23/23	23/23	18/2
Malignant glioma	17/17	17/17	6/17	1/1
Fibrillary astrocytoma	8/8	8/8	4/8	0
Astrocytoma	7/7	7/7	5/7	1/7
Mixed astrocytoma	1/1	1/1	1/1	0
Ganglioglioma	1/1	1/1	1/1	1/1
Gliofibroma	1/1		1/1	0
Medulloepithelioma	2/2	2/2	1/2	0
Hemangioblastoma	1/1	1/1	1/1	0
Lymphoma	1/1		1/1	0
Malignant teratoma			1/1	0
Ependymoma	8/10	6/10	9/10	0

[a] Signal intensity change relative to that of normal grey matter.

Table 4. MR characteristics of specific histologic types of tumors

	T2WI
Isointense to cortex	
PNET	40/42
Gliofibroma	1/1
Lymphoma	1/1
Mixed signal intensity	
Ependymoma	4/10
Malignant teratoma	1/1

tumors with the exception of the pilocytic astrocytomas (18/23 = 78.3% cystic) (fig. 3c), the ganglioglioma (1/1 = 100%), the astrocytomas (1/7 = 14.3%) and the malignant gliomas (1/17 = 5.9%) (table 3). In two instances the PNET presented as an acutely hemorrhagic mass (1-day-old male, 10-year-old male) in which the signal characteristics on T2WI were those of deoxyhemoglobin, markedly hypointense (fig. 4). In both instances, nonhemorrhagic tumor could not be seen separate from the area of acute hemorrhage. No other tumors in this series presented as acute hemorrhages.

Thus, the PNET can be best separated from other tumors by its common location in the cerebellum and its relative isointensity to grey matter on T2WI (fig. 1). The lack of cyst formation and the presence of contrast enhancement, while both commonly present in the

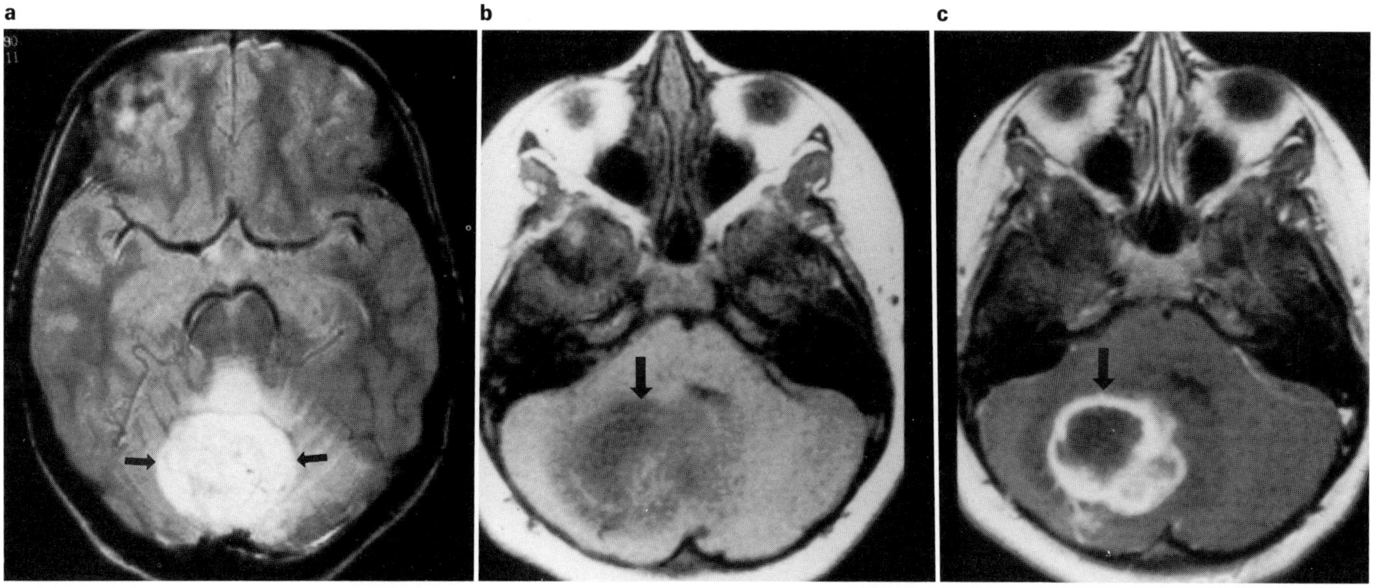

Fig. 2. Pilocytic cerebellar astrocytoma. **a** Axial T2WI on a 10-year-old male shows a high signal intensity mass (arrow) in the vermis. **b** Axial T1WI of a 6-year-old male show a hypointense mass (arrow) in the right cerebellar hemisphere, compressing the 4th ventricle and displacing it to the left. **c** Axial T1WI postgadolinium injection (same patient as **b**) shows ring-like contrast enhancement of the tumor (arrow).

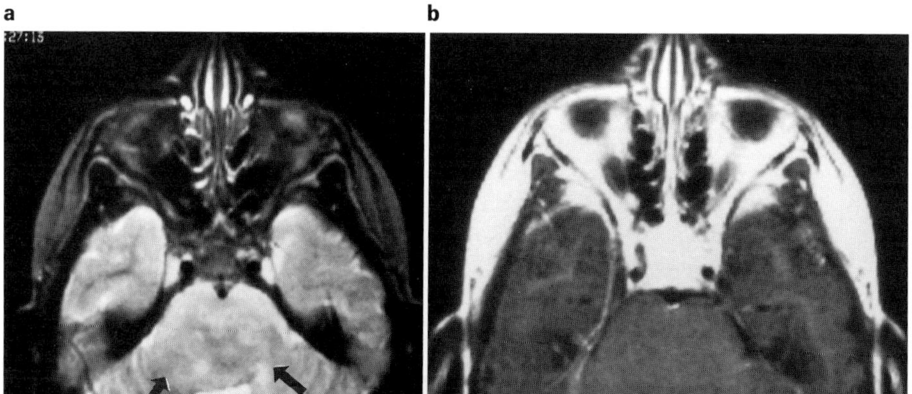

Fig. 3. Malignant brainstem glioma. **a** Axial T2WI shows a high signal intensity mass (arrows) expanding the pons, with more mass effect on the right side of the 4th ventricle. **b** Axial T1WI postgadolinium injection shows no evidence of contrast enhancement within the pontine mass.

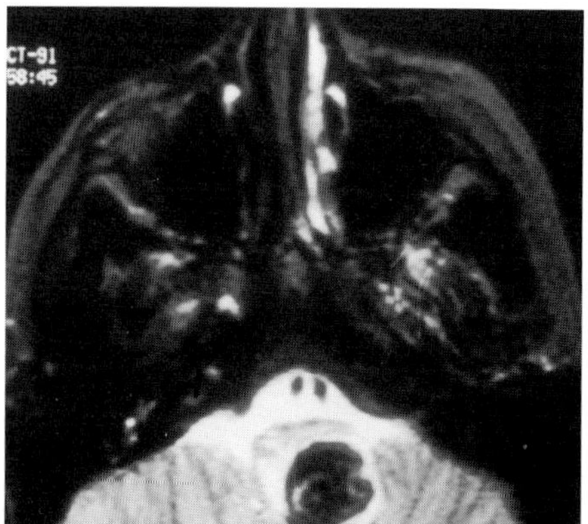

Fig. 4. Hemorrhagic primitive neuroectodermal tumor of the medulla. Axial T2WI in a 10-year-old male shows marked hypointensity of deoxyhemoglobin (arrow) within the medulla at the site of hemorrhage within the PNET.

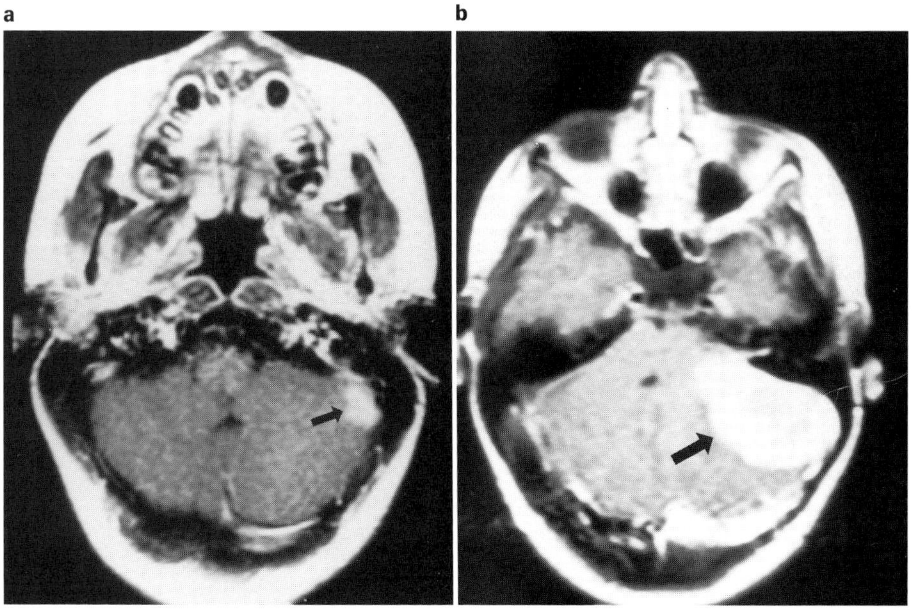

Fig. 5. Rapidly growing PNET. **a** Axial T1WI postgadolinium injection shows a small area of contrast enhancement (arrow) in the lateral aspect of the left cerebellar hemisphere in an 8-year-old female. **b** Axial T1WI postgadolinium injection 8 weeks later shows a large lateral cerebellar hemispheric contrast-enhanced tumor.

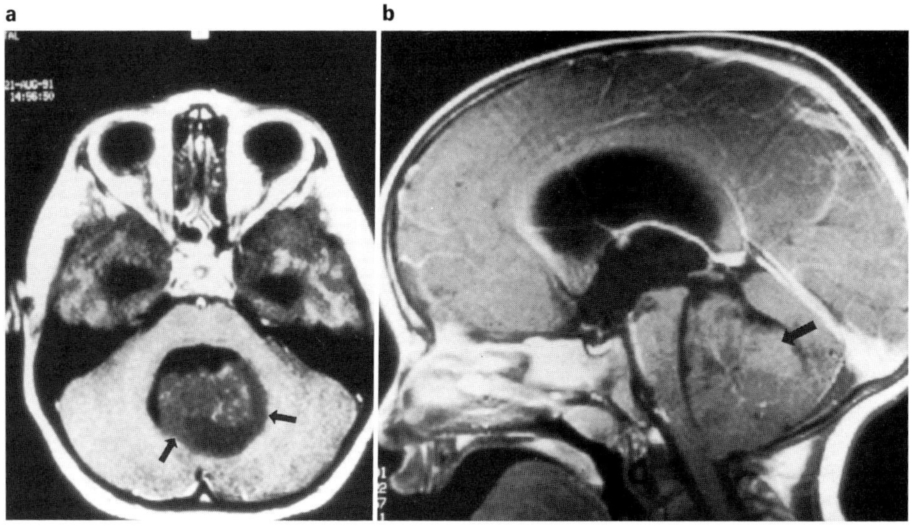

Fig. 6. Nonenhancing posterior fossa tumors (PNET, ependymoma). **a** Axial T1WI postgadolinium injection shows a large tumor mass (arrows) projecting into the 4th ventricle from the vermis. This mass does not enhance other than for a few vessels within the mass. **b** Sagittal T1WI postgadolinium injection shows a large mass (arrow) within the 4th ventricle that does not enhance except for several vessels within the mass.

PNET, are not specific. However, the presence of a cyst is useful in distinguishing commonly cystic cerebellar astrocytomas from the PNET. Problems that were encountered in making the initial diagnosis of PNET occurred in the 2 patients that presented as acute hematomas, so that the PNET should enter the differential diagnosis of an acute brainstem (fig. 4) or cerebellar bleed. Also, both the gliofibroma and the lymphoma of the posterior fossa were not distinguishable from the PNETs by signal intensity or MR enhancement.

A further problem was encountered in 1 patient, when on a study performed for follow-up of a supratentorial abnormality, a small area of contrast enhancement was demonstrated in the lateral aspected of the cerebellar hemisphere (fig. 5a). This was reported as a suspicious area that could represent a very small tumor, but could also represent other disease processes. Eight weeks later the mass was much larger (fig. 5b) and the patient was symptomatic from the rapidly growing posterior fossa PNET.

In 2 patients where the PNET did not enhance (2/22 = 9%) (fig. 6a), this finding necessitated inclusion in the differential diagnosis of the equally common nonenhancing ependymoma (1/10 = 10%) (table 3) (fig. 6b). The ependymomas were the most common tumor to initially present as an intra-4th ventricular mass (10/11 = 90.9%).

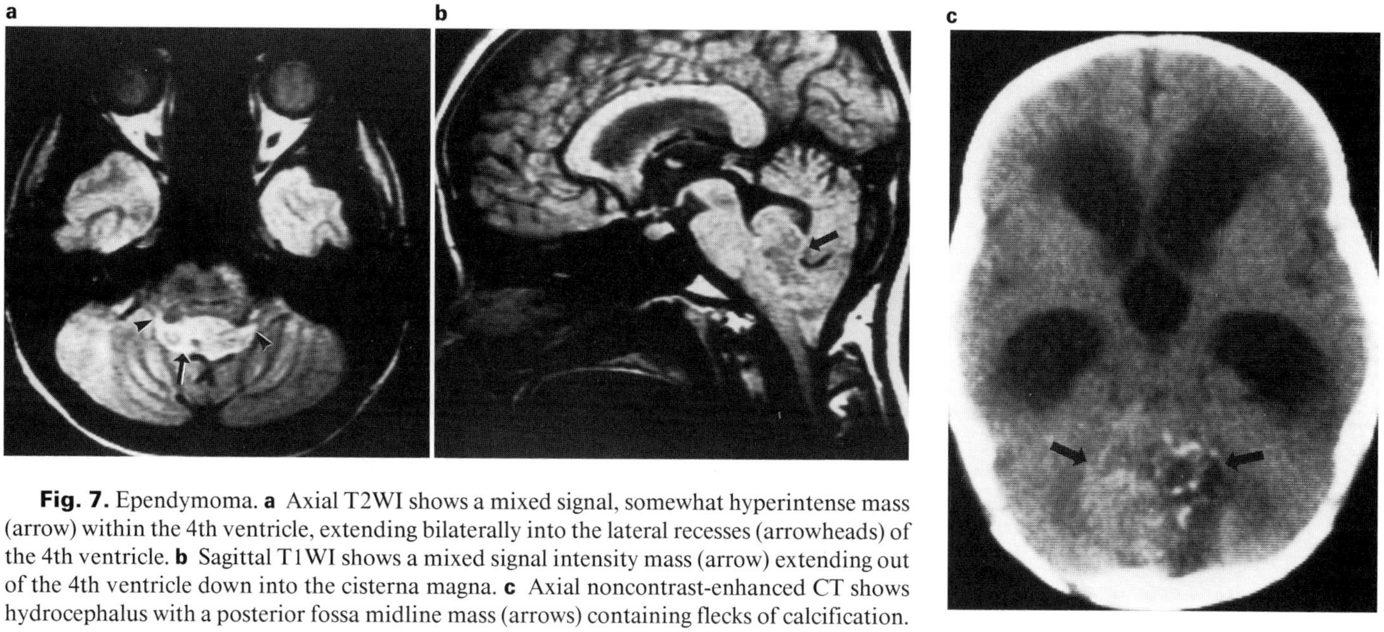

Fig. 7. Ependymoma. **a** Axial T2WI shows a mixed signal, somewhat hyperintense mass (arrow) within the 4th ventricle, extending bilaterally into the lateral recesses (arrowheads) of the 4th ventricle. **b** Sagittal T1WI shows a mixed signal intensity mass (arrow) extending out of the 4th ventricle down into the cisterna magna. **c** Axial noncontrast-enhanced CT shows hydrocephalus with a posterior fossa midline mass (arrows) containing flecks of calcification.

Their typical extension into the cerebellopontine angle through the lateral recesses of the 4th ventricle was demonstrated (fig. 7a), although exophytic cerebellar and brainstem astrocytomas involving in part the inferior or middle cerebellar peduncles can mimic the appearance of an ependymoma within the lateral recess. The ependymoma was the tumor that most often had a heterogenous signal intensity on the T1WI (2/10 = 20%) and T2WI (4/10 = 40%) (table 4; fig. 7b). This appeared to reflect the contribution to signal intensity from dystrophic calcification, hemorrhage of various ages and small areas of tumor necrosis. Calcification is poorly seen, if at all, on MR, and CT remains the imaging procedure of choice in its demonstration. Thc presence of small flecks of calcification on CT has been reported in up to 50% of posterior fossa ependymomas [4] (fig. 7c), but in only 15% of PNETs [5] and 20% of cerebellar astrocytomas [6], indicating that CT may have a roll in helping in the differential diagnosis when MR findings do not resolve the issue.

Among pitfalls in this series was a case in which it was difficult to differentiate a laterally placed ependymoma from an astrocytoma involving the cerebellar peduncle and another case with an astrocytoma of the cerebellar peduncle (fig. 8) in which the ependymoma remained a preoperative diagnostic consideration.

The brainstem and cerebellar astrocytomas and gliomas were most often low in signal on T1WI (57/57 = 100%) and high on T2WI (57/57 = 100%) (table 3; fig. 3a). This combination of signal intensity changes, similar to that seen in supratentorial gliomas and astrocytomas in both children and adults, serves to distinguish these tumors from the isointense to gray matter PNET on T2WI and from the occasionally mixed signal intensity ependymoma. While the initial absence of contrast enhancement in pontine tumors (fig. 3b) was associated

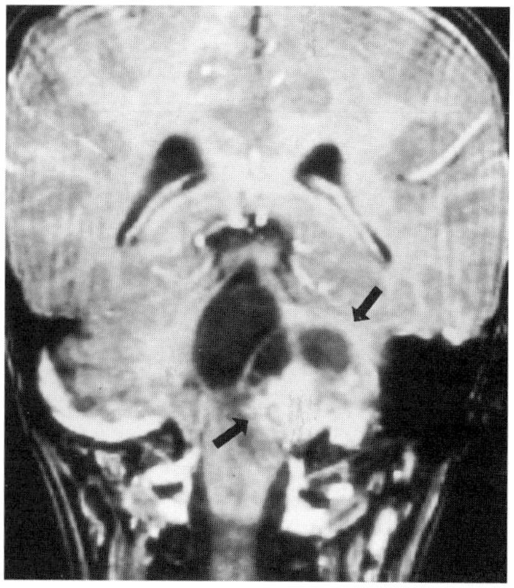

Fig. 8. Pilocytic astrocytoma of the inferior cerebellar peduncle mimicking ependymoma of the cerebellopontine angle. Coronal T1WI, fat-saturated, postgadolinium injection shows an enhanced tumor mass (arrows) in the lateral recess of the 4th ventricle. The 4th ventricle appears dilated and free of tumor.

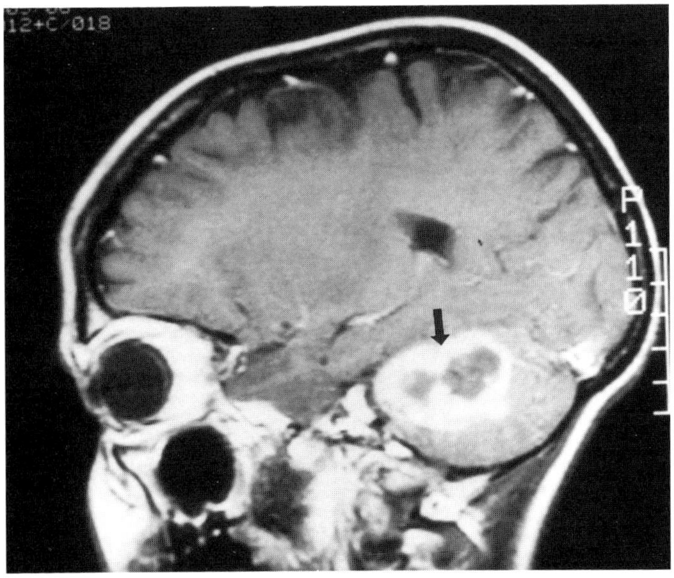

Fig. 9. Glioblastoma cerebellum. Sagittal T1WI postgadolinium injection shows contrast enhancement of a cerebellar hemispheric centrally necrotic mass (arrow) in a patient 10 years postradiation therapy for lymphoma.

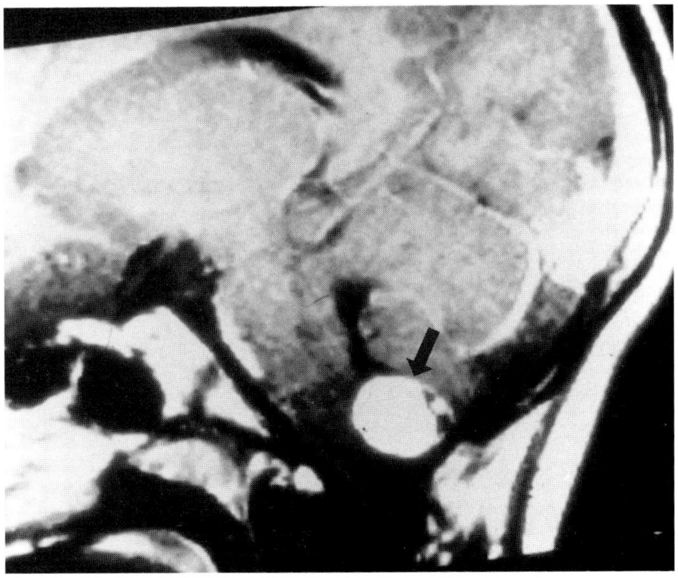

Fig. 10. Hemangioblastoma medulla oblongata (von Hippel Lindau syndrome). Sagittal T1WI postgadolinium injection shows contrast enhancement of an exophytic mass (arrow) arising from the medulla oblongata in a 10-year-old female who has had prior resection of an ocular hemangioblastoma.

with the likelihood of a subsequent diagnosis of malignancy (11/13 = 84.6%), the presence of contrast enhancement usually did signify a benign cerebellar (26/30 = 86.6%) tumor (table 3; fig. 2b). In three of the four malignant cerebellar gliomas (fig. 9) there was a prior history of radiation therapy (2 for treatment of prior PNET and 1 for treatment of lymphoma). Such a history should alert the physician to the likelihood of these tumors being secondary to radiation therapy and more aggressive. The one cerebellar ganglioglioma was indistinguishable on the basis of MR imaging from either the low grade astrocytomas or malignant gliomas of the cerebellum.

Diagnostic problems were encountered in three cases of intrinsic brainstem masses. In one instance a hemorrhagic PNET (fig. 4) could not be distinguished from a spontaneous bleed of other etiology. In another instance, a pontine tumor that had all the MR findings associated with a brainstem glioma proved at autopsy to be a medulloepithelioma. A misdiagnosis also occurred in the case of a cerebellar medulloepithelioma when the imaging characteristics were similar to that of an astrocytoma. In the third instance a contrast-enhancing exophytic medullary tumor (fig. 10) that had the appearance of a brainstem glioma proved to be a hemangioblastoma at surgery. In the hemangioblastoma case, a correct preoperative diagnosis was made, not on the imaging findings, but on the basis of the clinical history of past resection of a retinal hemangioblastoma and the clinical suspicion of Von Hippel Lindau syndrome.

References

1 Gusnard DA: Cerebellar neoplasms in children. Semin Roentgenol 1990;25:263–278.
2 Smith RR: Brain stem tumors. Semin Roentgenol 1990;25:249–262.
3 Zimmerman RA: Pediatric supratentorial tumors. Semin Roentgenol 1990;25:225–248.
4 Swartz JD, Zimmerman RA, Bilaniuk LT: Computed tomography of intracranial ependymomas. Radiology 1982;143:97–101.
5 Zimmerman RA, Bilaniuk LT, Pahlajani H: Spectrum of medulloblastomas demonstrated by computed tomography. Radiology 1978; 126:137–141.
6 Zimmerman RA, Bilaniuk LT, Bruno L, et al: Computed tomography of cerebellar astrocytoma. AJR 1978;130:929–933.

Pediatr Neurosurg 1992;18:65–83

A. James Barkovich
Michael S.B. Edwards

Neuroradiology Section, Department of Radiology and Division of Pediatric Neurosurgery, University of California, San Francisco, Calif., USA

Applications of Neuroimaging in Hydrocephalus

Key Words
Hydrocephalus
Magnetic resonance imaging
Computerized tomography
Cerebrospinal fluid

Abstract
Hydrocephalus is a common problem in pediatric neurological and neurosurgical practices. In this manuscript, the common imaging appearances of hydrocephalus are discussed in relation to the underyling causes of the hydrocephalus. Moreover, specific findings seen on magnetic resonance imaging (MR) examinations are discussed and contrasted with those on computed x-ray tomography (CT) and ultrasound. Finally the imaging findings associated with treatment of hydrocephalus are discussed. In particular, analysis of shunt function, the diagnosis of shunt failure, and the complications of shunting are stressed.

Radiographic Diagnosis of Hydrocephalus

The radiologic diagnosis of hydrocephalus has evolved with the increasing sophistication of imaging modalities. Classically, the diagnosis was made on skull films by the presence of split sutures, increased craniofacial ratio, bulging of the anterior fontanelle, and, occasionally, a 'hammered silver' appearance when the hydrocephalus was chronic. Ultrasound, computed x-ray tomography (CT), and magnetic resonance imaging (MR) are much more sensitive than plain radiographs in the detection of hydrocephalus. The diagnosis of hydrocephalus is made when the ventricles are enlarged in the absence of atrophy. However, the differentiation of ventricular enlargement secondary to hydrocephalus and that resulting from white matter atrophy is not always easy; the differentiation is particularly difficult in the pediatric population. Several parameters have therefore been devised to aid in this determination. The parameters that favor hydrocephalus include: (1) commensurate dilatation of the temporal horn with the lateral ventricles, (2) enlargement of the anterior or posterior recesses of the third ventricle, (3) narrowing of the mammilopontine distance, (4) narrowing of the ventricular angle, (5) widening of the frontal horn radius, and (6) effacement of cortical sulci (fig. 1). It has also been suggested that an accentuated cerebrospinal fluid (CSF) 'flow-void' (that is, loss of signal of CSF) is seen in the third ventricle, aqueduct of Sylvius, and fourth ventricle of hydrocephalic patients as a result of hyperdynamic flow [9, 10]. Other authors, however, dispute the specificity of this finding [71].

The most reliable signs in the differentiation of hydrocephalus from the ex vacuo ventricular enlargement of white matter atrophy are *commensurate dilatation of the temporal horns* with the bodies of the lateral ventricles (fig. 2A, B) [37–45] and *enlargement of the anterior and posterior recesses of the third ventricle* [2, 18] (fig. 2A, C, 3), both of which strongly suggest hydrocephalus. Several

A. James Barkovich, MD
Neuroradiology Section, L371
Department of Radiology
University of California, San Francisco
San Francisco, CA 94143–0625 (USA)

1016–2291/92/0182–0065
$2.75/0

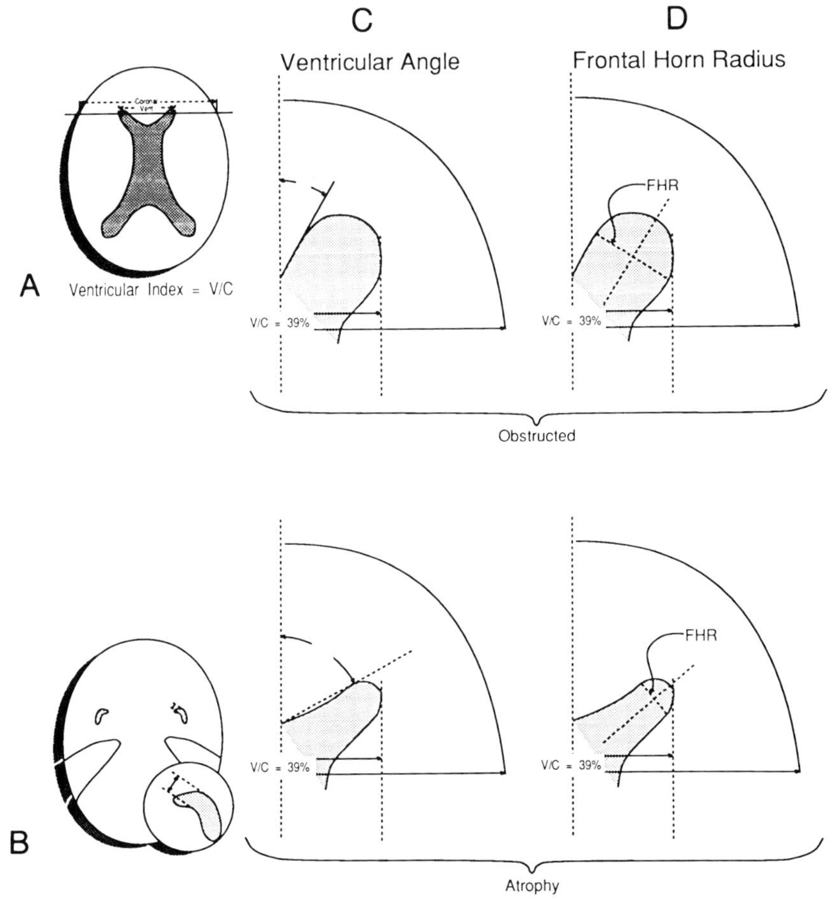

Fig. 1. Various methods in the radiographic diagnosis of hydrocephalus. **A** The ventricular index is the ratio of the ventricular diameter at the level of the frontal horns to the diameter of the brain measured at the same level. This is not a very sensitive or specific measurement in the detection of hydrocephalus because the ventricular index enlarged in cerebral atrophy as well as in hydrocephalus. **B** Enlargement of the temporal horns commensurately with the bodies of the lateral ventricles is probably the most sensitive and reliable sign in the differentiation of hydrocephalus from atrophy. There is significantly less dilatation of the temporal horns than the bodies of the lateral ventricles in cerebral atrophy. **C** The ventricular angle measures the divergence of the frontal horn. In theory, the angle made by the anterior or superior margins of the frontal horn at the level of the foramina of Monro is diminished when concentric enlargement of the frontal horns occurs. Compare the illustration of hydrocephalus (top) with that of atrophy (bottom). The ventricular index in both instances is 39%; however, the ventricular angle is markedly reduced in hydrocephalus. **D** The frontal horn radius (FHR) measures the widest diameter of the frontal horns taken at a 90° angle to the long axis of the frontal horn. The usefulness of this measurement is demonstrated by the markedly increased frontal horn radius in the patient with hydrocephalus (top) as opposed to the patient with atrophy (bottom). Overall, no one measurement is completely accurate in the diagnosis of hydrocephalus; the size of the temporal horns, ventricular angle, the frontal horn radius, and the size of the ventricles as compared to the cortical sulci should all be assessed [from 2, with permission].

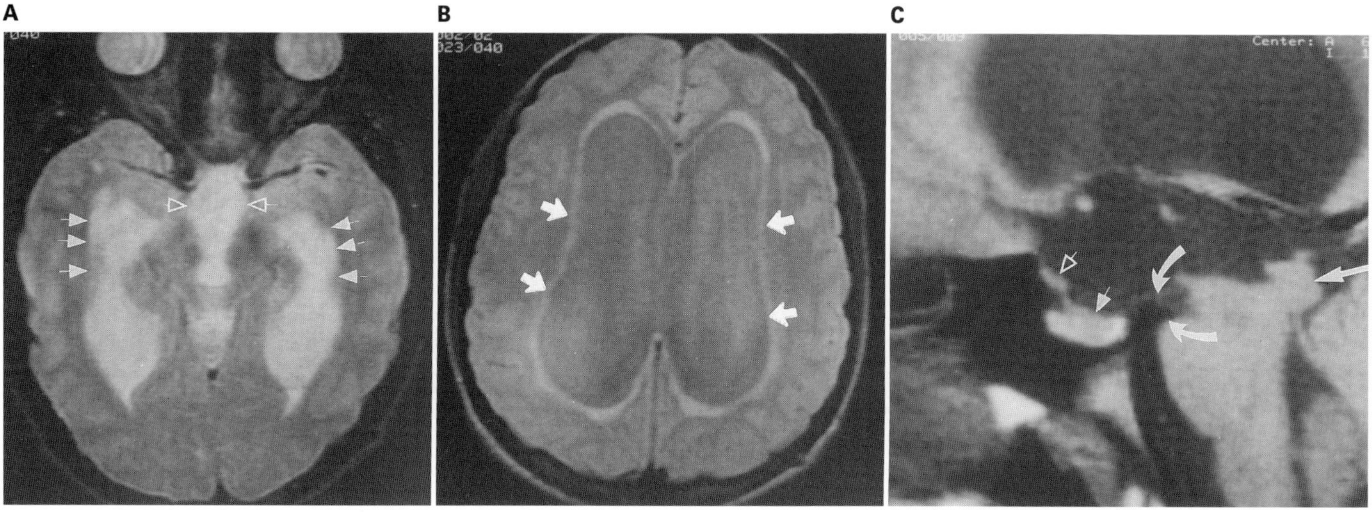

Fig. 2. MR findings in hydrocephalus. **A** Axial T2-weighted image at the level of the third ventricle and temporal horns shows dilated anterior recesses (open arrows) of the third ventricle and temporal horns of the lateral ventricles (closed arrows). **B** Axial T2-weighted image (first echo) shows lateral ventricles (arrows) that are dilated commensurately with the temporal horns in **A**. **C** Sagittal T1-weighted image shows massive dilatation of the anterior recesses of the third ventricle. The chiasmatic recess (open arrow) and infundibular recess (closed arrow) are both markedly dilated. In addition, the mammilopontine distance (curved arrows) is reduced. Note that the quadrigeminal plate (long arrow) is compressed in the superior-inferior plane by the dilated suprapineal recess.

studies have shown that there is significantly less dilatation of the temporal horns than the bodies of the lateral ventricles in cerebral atrophy [37, 72]. The reason for the discrepancy in ventricular enlargement between the temporal lobe and the frontal, parietal and occipital lobes is not fully understood; however, the rather small size of the temporal lobes and, in particular, the relatively small volume of white matter in the temporal lobes may play a role [45]. The reason for the disproportionate enlargement of the recesses of the third ventricle is presumably the simple fact that no brain tissue borders the ventricle at those regions, diminishing the resistance to ventricular expansion under conditions of increased intraventricular pressure. Enlargement of the anterior (chiasmal and infundibular) recesses seems to occur earlier and more severely than enlargement of the posterior (suprapineal) recess [18]. Diminution of the *mammillopontine distance* is related to the enlargement of the anterior third ventricular recesses in that it is caused by downward displacement of the floor of the third ventricle (fig. 2C).

The *ventricular angle* (fig. 1) measures the divergence of the frontal horns. The angle between the anterior or superior margins of the frontal horns at the level of the foramina of Monro is diminished by concentric enlargement of the frontal horns [37]. The diminution of the angle may be appreciated on either axial or coronal images. The concentric enlargement of the frontal horns eventually produces the so-called 'Mickey Mouse ears' image on axial scans. This concentric enlargement of the frontal horns also causes enlargement of the so-called *frontal horn radius* (fig. 1) which is determined by measuring the widest diameter of the frontal horns taken at a 90° angle to the long axis of the frontal horn [37]. The final indicator of hydrocephalus is enlargement of the ventricular system to a degree that *is disproportionate to the enlargement of the cortical sulci* [45]. The theory behind this parameter is that increasing pressure within the ventricular system causes compression of the brain tissue against the inner table of the skull and consequent diminution of sulcal size. In pediatric patients, however, this parameter is often misleading because either atrophy or hydrocepalus can enlarge both the ventricles and sulci [28]. Further complicating the radiologic assessment is the fact that the size of the ventricles and subarachnoid spaces is quite variable over the first 2 years of life [43].

In view of the fact that both atrophy and hydrocephalus can cause enlargement of both ventricles and cortical sulci, complicated by a wide variation in the normal ventricular size of infants, imaging studies alone are sometimes not adequate to differentiate hydrocephalus from atrophy [2, 28]. A large or enlarging head indicates hydro-

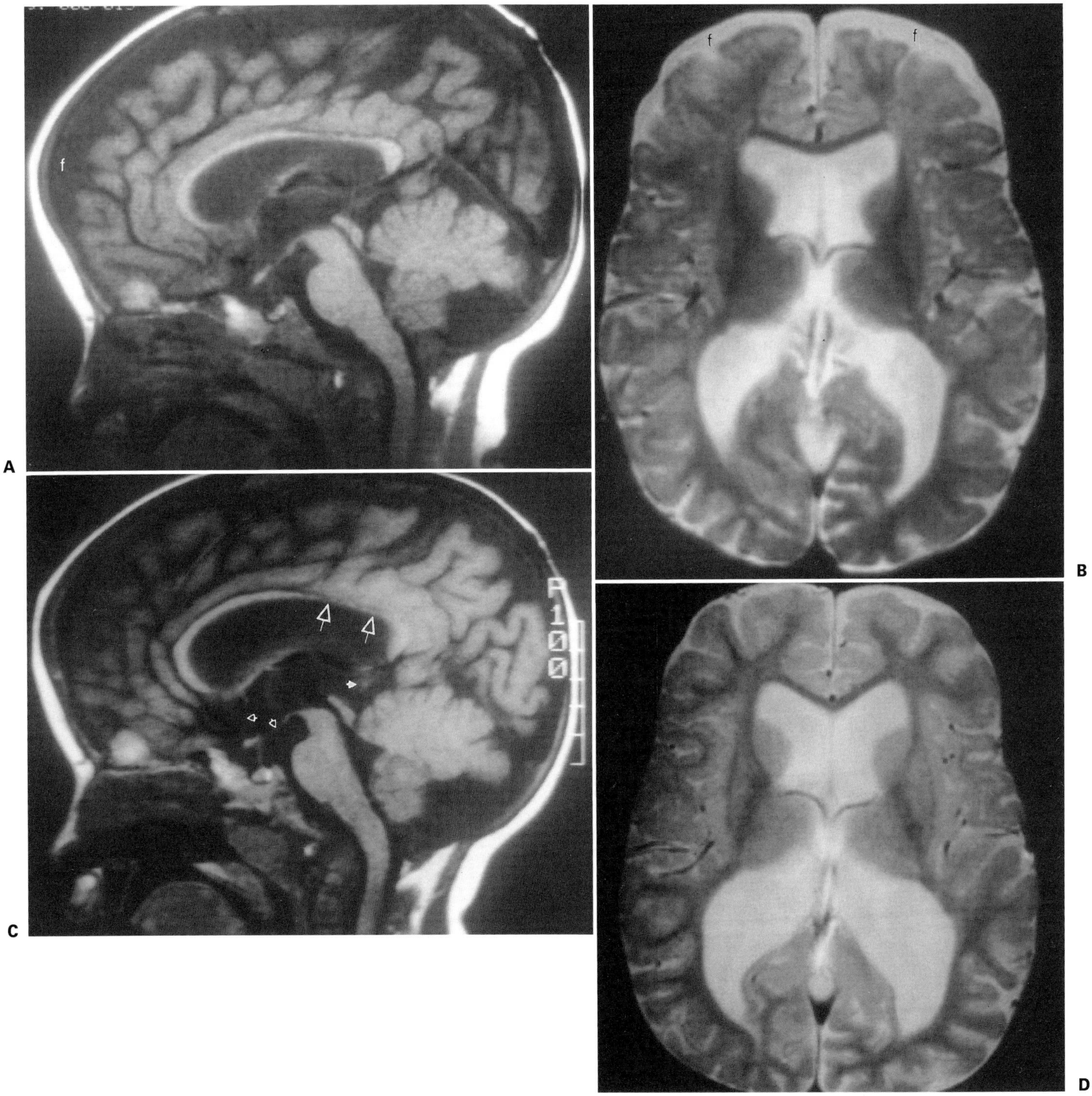

Fig. 3. Use of third ventricular recesses in the diagnosis of hydrocephalus. Infant with macrocephaly. **A, B** Sagittal T1 and axial T2 weighted images in a 6-month-old show large ventricles with large extra-axial fluid collections (f). Third ventricular recesses are equivocal. Differential diagnosis was benign subdural collections of infancy versus mild hydrocephalus. **C, D** Follow-up scans 1 year later show diminished size of the extra-axial fluid. However, the anterior and inferior walls (open arrows) of the third ventricle and the posterior recess (closed arrow) of the third ventricle are now definitely bowed outward, and the aqueduct is enlarged, establishing the diagnosis of hydrocephalus.

cephalus whereas a small or diminishing head circumference is more compatible with atrophy. Monitoring of intracranial pressure is another important factor in the differentiation of hydrocephalus from atrophy. Radionuclide flow studies with technetium-99m DTPA may be useful [35, 40]. Patients with extraventricular obstructive hydrocephalus may demonstrate reflux of the radionuclide into the ventricles with a delay in flow over the convexities. Normally, flow should extend over the convexities within 24 h [35, 40].

The finding of interstitial edema resulting from transependymal flow of CSF is a further radiological finding that may be helpful in the diagnosis of hydrocephalus, particularly in children. When pressure within the ventricular system is increased, CSF enters the extracellular spaces of the the brain through the ependymal lining of the ventricles. CSF then flows through the brain parenchyma to the arachnoid villi or other sites of CSF absorption. The consequent increased water within the cerebral parenchyma can be detected both on CT and MR. On CT, it appears as hypodensity in the periventricular region. On MR, the increase in water appears as a rim of prolonged T1 and T2 relaxation times surrounding the lateral ventricles (fig. 2B). This rim is often not appreciated on the long TR/TE sequences because the rim of high signal intensity blends in with the CSF within the ventricle; a long TR, short TE ('proton density') image is much more sensitive.

Although the parameters described in the preceding paragraphs are sometimes helpful in the diagnosis of hydrocephalus and in the differentiation of obstructive hydrocephalus from atrophy, in practice, the diagnosis of hydrocephalus remains largely intuitive. In general, diffuse enlargement of the lateral ventricles with commensurate temporal horn enlargement (in the absence of significant enlargement of the sylvian fissures or other evidence of temporal lobe atrophy), enlargement of the anterior recesses of the third ventricle, and a general rounding of the frontal horn shape in the proper clinical setting indicate hydrocephalus.

Distortions of Brain and Ventricular System Resulting from Hydrocephalus

Severe hydrocephalus may cause herniation of portions of the ventricular system or distortion of the adjacent brain. Such herniations and distortions can cause confusion in the interpretation of imaging studies and will therefore be discussed as a separate section.

A common distortion resulting from severe hydrocephalus is the formation of atrial diverticula (fig. 4, 5), herniations of the ventricular wall through the choroidal fissure of the ventricular trigone into the supracerebellar and quadrigeminal cisterns [56]. These diverticula can compress the mesencephalic tectum and can be mistaken for arachnoid cysts in the region of the quadrigeminal cistern (fig. 4). Coronal images are very helpful in the evaluation of these patients since they often demonstrate the continuity of the trigone of the lateral ventricle with the diverticulum.

The suprapineal recess of the third ventricle is another common site of ventricular herniation. The dilated recess expands into the posterior incisural space, displacing the pineal gland inferiorly and occasionally elevating the vein of Galen. Large diverticula can extend inferiorly to compress the quadrigeminal plate. Such compression can cause a shortening of the tectum in the rostral-caudal direction (fig. 2C) [4]. Such a shortened, thickened tectum should not be mistaken for a neoplasm; isointensity of the tectum with normal brain tissue on long TR/TE images excludes a tumor. A dilated suprapineal recess may also extend inferiorly, posterior to the quadrigeminal plate, to compress the plate in the anterior-posterior dimension, resulting in thinning of the tectum and narrowing of the aqueduct [4].

The anterior recesses of the third ventricle (the chiasmal and infundibular recesses) can enlarge and extend inferiorly into the suprasellar cistern in patients with moderate to severe hydrocephalus (fig. 4A). The enlargement and inferior displacement of these recesses can compress the infundibulum and diminish flow within the hypothalamic-pituitary portal venous system, resulting in hypothalamic-pituitary dysfunction [42]. These enlarged anterior recesses and their pulsations may erode the dorsum sellae, one of the classic plain film findings in hydrocephalus.

When communicating hydrocephalus is severe, the cerebral hemispheres and temporal lobes in particular can enlarge markedly, narrowing the quadrigeminal cistern. In some patients, the enlarged temporal lobes may compress the quadrigeminal plate, causing a moulding of the tectum and a secondary compression of the aqueduct (fig. 5). In such patients, the question may arise as to whether the hydrocephalus may be primarily communicating in nature with aqueductal narrowing being a secondary phenomenon [4, 8, 76].

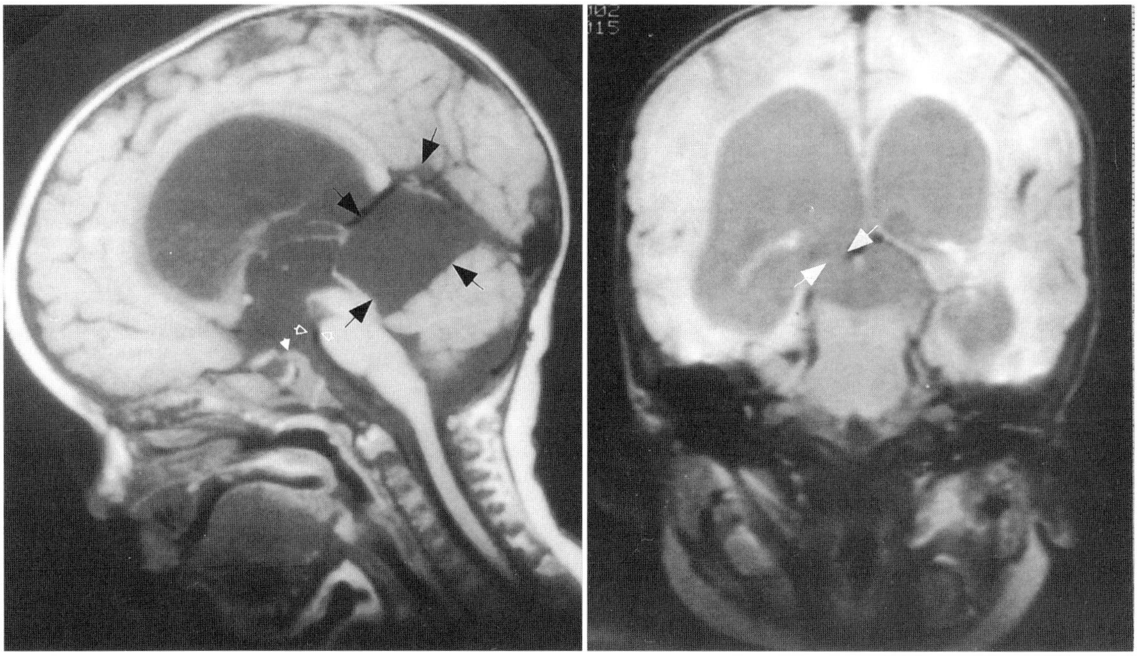

A B

Fig. 4. Hydrocephalus with atrial diverticulum mimicking a quadrigeminal cistern cyst. **A** Sagittal T1-weighted image shows severe hydrocephalus. Note the marked dilatation of the anterior recesses of the third ventricle, narrowing the mammilopontine distance (open white arrows) and eroding the dorsum sellae (closed white arrow). A large cyst (black arrows) is seen posterior to the quadrigeminal plate, compressing the plate and narrowing the inferior aqueduct. **B** Coronal image shows continuity of the atrium of the right lateral ventricle with the cyst through the choroidal fissure (arrows). The retrotectal cyst disappeared after a ventriculoperitoneal shunt was placed [from 2, with permission].

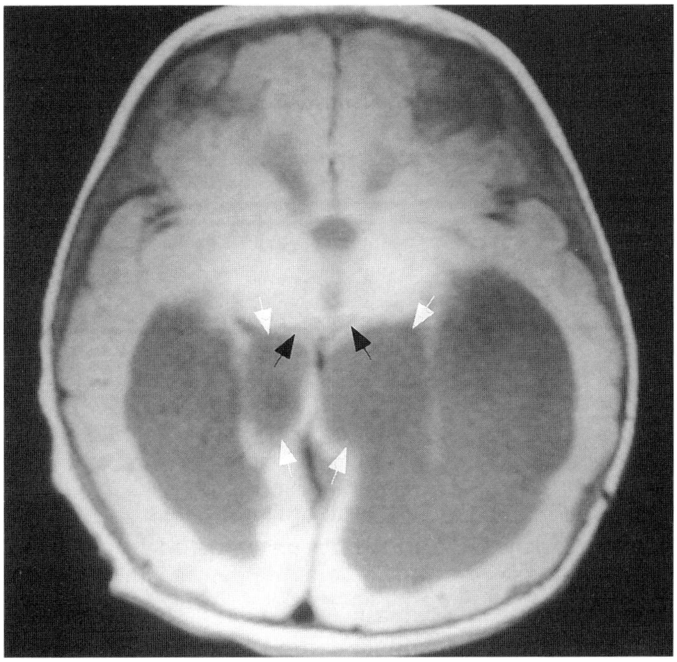

Fig. 5. Hydrocephalus with atrial diverticula compressing tectum. Axial T1-weighted image shows the bilateral atrial diverticula (white arrows) compressing and distorting the tectum (black arrows).

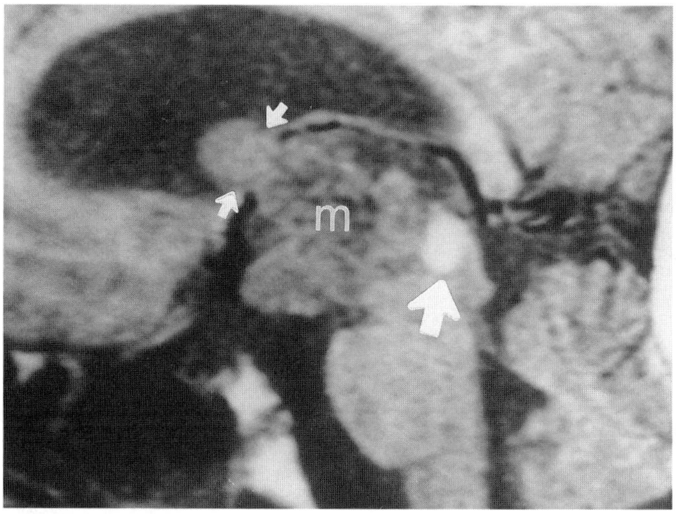

Fig. 6. Residual craniopharyngioma blocking foramina of Monro and cerebral aqueduct. A large mass (m) sits in the third ventricle, extending through the foramen of Monro (small arrows) into the lateral ventricle and extending into the proximal aqueduct (large arrows).

Specific Categories of Hydrocephalus

Both hydrocephalus secondary to overproduction of CSF and hydrocephalus secondary to disturbances of normal CSF flow and absorption are evaluated well by CT and MR imaging and by ultrasonography in young infants with large fontanelles. Noncommunicating (intraventricular obstructive) hydrocephalus, however, is probably best evaluated by MR. The reason for the superiority of MR is that the increased contrast resolution and the ability to image in three planes allows better differentiation of subtle mass lesions from webs, membranes, and stenoses.

Another advantage of MR is the ability to qualitatively and quantitatively assess CSF flow [20, 46, 61, 70]. On routine spin-echo MR scans, dynamic CSF flow can be detected by signal loss in areas of rapid or turbulent flow [9, 70]. By manipulating parameters, rapidly moving CSF can be made to appear bright while keeping the signal of stationary or slowly flowing CSF dark; the patency of the aqueduct can be assessed in this way [1]. Finally, special techniques that take advantage of the change in phase angle of moving spins can be used to quantitate the flow of CSF through the foramina of Monro, aqueduct, foramen of Magendie, or brainstem cisterns [20].

Hydrocephalus Resulting from Excessive Formation of CSF (Choroid Plexus Papillomas)

Choroid plexus papillomas are easily diagnosed on both CT and MR by their characteristic location and appearance. On CT, choroid plexus *papillomas* are isodense or mildly hyperdense to normal brain with occasional punctate foci of calcification. The mass is usually situated at the trigone but may be located anywhere along the choroid plexus and into the frontal horn and third ventricle. Rarely, the tumor may originate in the fourth ventricle or in the cerebellopontine angle [50]. Homogeneous enhancement is seen after infusion of intravenous contrast [15, 27, 58]. On MR, choroid plexus *papillomas* are lobulated intraventricular masses that tend to be homogeneous on both short TR and long TR sequences and are characteristically hypointense on long TR images [3, 15]. Foci of hemorrhage or calcium can occasionally be seen within the tumor.

Hydrocephalus Secondary to Intraventricular Obstruction of CSF Flow (Noncommunicating Hydrocephalus)

Mass Lesions

Noncommunicating hydrocephalus may result from any obstruction of the ventricular system from the lateral ventricles to the foramina of Magendie and Luschka. Tumors and cysts are the most common cause of noncommunicating hydrocephalus in the pediatric age group.

Masses can grow into and obstruct the foramina of Monro from a number of directions. Tumors originating in the lateral ventricles, such as ependymomas, astrocytomas, or meningiomas, and tumors originating in the third ventricle, such as astrocytomas, choroid plexus papillomas, teratomas, or, rarely, craniopharyngiomas (fig. 6) can grow into and obstruct the foramina of Monro. Suprasellar tumors and cysts may occasionally grow upward to the foramina, pushing the floor of the third ventricle superiorly. In patient with tuberous sclerosis, giant cell astrocytomas which originate adjacent to the foramina of Monro, often grow medially into the foramina to produce an obstruction.

Obstruction of the sylvian aqueduct is a common cause of hydrocephalus. A common cause of obstruction at this level in children is a tumor of the pineal region. Germ cell tumors (germinoma, endodermal sinus tumor, embryonal cell carcinoma, choriocarcinoma, teratoma), tumors of pineal origin (pineocytoma, pineoblastoma),

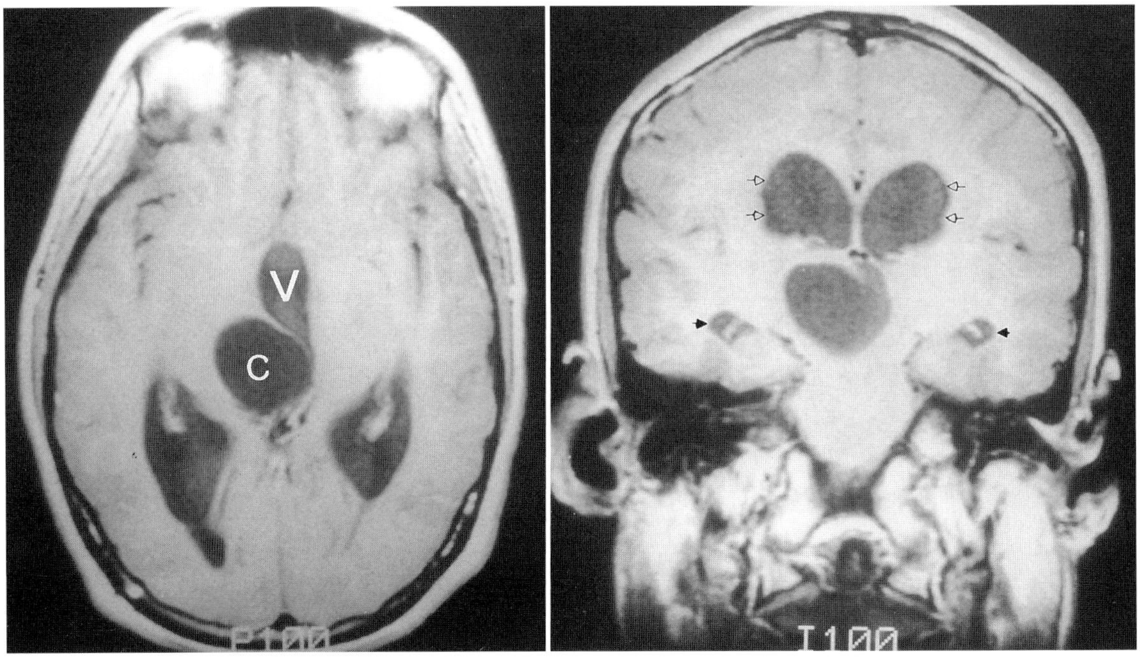

A B

Fig. 7. Neuroepithelial cyst. **A** Axial T1-weighted image shows a cyst (C) originating in the right thalamus and compressing the posterior third ventricle. The anterior third ventricle (V) is enlarged. **B** Coronal T1-weighted image shows enlargement of the ventricular bodies (open arrows) and temporal horns (closed arrows).

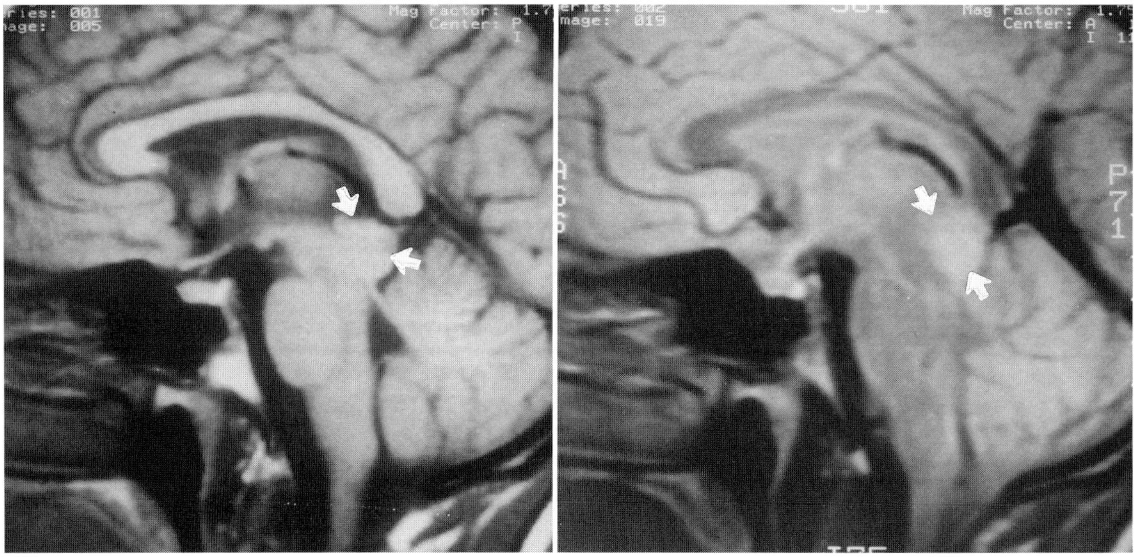

A B

Fig. 8. Tectal glioma. **A** Sagittal T1-weighted image shows a mass (arrows) involving the quadrigeminal plate and narrowing the aqueduct. The lateral and third ventricles are normal in size because a ventriculoperitoneal shunt has been placed. **B** Sagittal T2-weighted image shows that the tumor (arrows) is hyperintense (has a long T2 relaxation time).

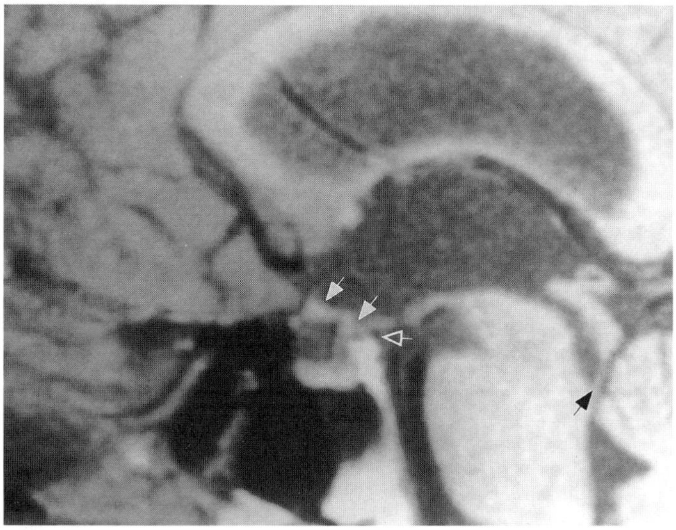

Fig. 9. Aqueductal web. Sagittal T1-weighted image shows a small slip of tissue (black arrow) stretched across the distal aqueduct. The proximal protion of the aqueduct is slightly dilated. Note the dilated anterior recesses of the third ventricle (closed white arrows) and the possible erosion of the dorsum sellae (open white arrow) [From 2, with permission].

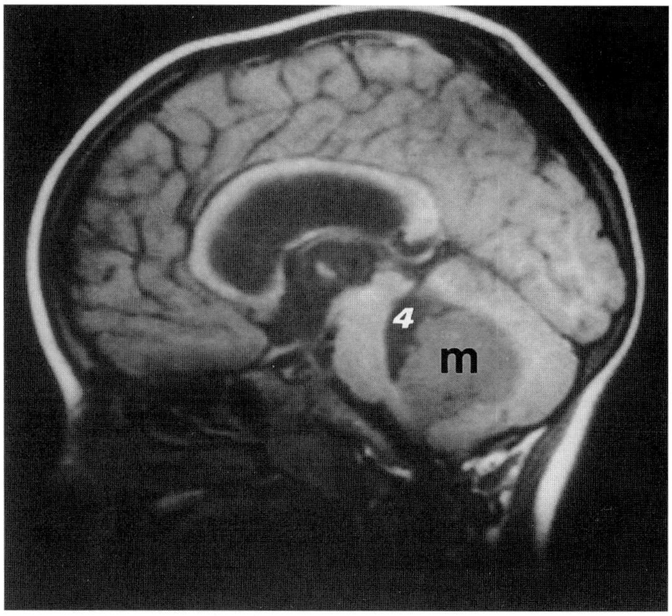

Fig. 10. Medulloblastoma. A large mass (m) is present in the fourth ventricle, obstructing CSF flow. Note the enlarged lateral and third ventricles and the expanded proximal fourth ventricle (4).

astrocytomas (from the thalami, quadrigeminal plate or the tegmentum of the midbrain), meningiomas (from the tentorium), tumors of the third ventricle (fig. 6), or varices of the vein of Galen may all present as a pineal region mass compressing the aqueduct. Neuroepithelial cysts originating in the thalami can grow posteromedially to obstruct the posterior third ventricle near the entrance to the aqueduct (fig. 7). Most of these lesions are easily identified by CT; however, astrocytomas of the quadrigeminal plate are often subtle and difficult to identify on CT. On MR, they are easily identified as bulbous tectal masses with prolonged T2 relaxation [3, 4] (fig. 8). Therefore, MR is essential to differentiate benign aqueductal stenosis (fig. 9) from stenosis secondary to a tectal astrocytoma in children with aqueductal stenosis.

Masses of the fourth ventricle and cerebellum frequently have caused hydrocephalus by the time of presentation. Imaging studies will show the posterior fossa mass blocking the flow of CSF out of the aqueduct and/or ventricle (fig. 10). Unlike cerebellar tumors, hydrocephalus is uncommonly present in patients with brain stem neoplasms.

Aqueductal Stenosis

The CT appearance of benign aqueductal stenosis is dilatation of the lateral and third ventricles with a normal sized fourth ventricle. This appearance may be misleading, however, since the fourth ventricle is normal in a large percentage of patients with communicating hydrocephalus. Moreover, as stated earlier, tectal astrocytomas that are large enough to obstruct the aqueduct can be missed on routine CT scans. In all patients with suspected aqueductal stenosis the posterior third ventricle should be carefully scrutinized for the presence of a mass. The MR findings in aqueductal stenosis are more specific but are nonetheless quite variable. Patients with severe hydrocephalus generally have a stenosis in the proximal aqueduct, either at the level of the superior colliculi or at the entrance to the aqueduct immediately inferior to the posterior commissure (fig. 4, 5) [4]. In patients with mild hydrocephalus, the level of obstruction is more often in the distal portion of the aqueduct. In patients with distal aqueductal stenosis, the proximal aqueduct tends to be dilated and the quadrigeminal plate is displaced posteriorly and stretched by the dilated proximal aqueduct (fig. 9). As stated previously, benign aqueductal stenosis and neoplastic aqueductal stenosis can be easily differentiated by MR in that tectal and tegmental gliomas that compress and obstruct the aqueduct appear as bulbous masses that have high signal intensity on long TR/TE images (fig. 8).

Aqueductal Gliosis

This is a postinflammatory process that is usually secondary to a perinatal infection or hemorrhage [65]. Aqueductal gliosis is becoming more prevalent as newborns with bacterial meningitis or intracranial hemorrhage survive at increasing rates. As in benign aqueductal stenosis, the onset of symptoms, which are those of hydrocephalus, is insidious. The ependymal lining of the aqueduct is destroyed and marked fibrillary gliosis of adjacent tissue is evident.

On imaging studies, differentiation of aqueductal stenosis from aqueductal gliosis is not possible. The appearance on both MR and CT is identical.

Congenital Anomalies

There are two major entities in this category. The more common entity is the *Chiari II malformation*, which accounts for approximately 40% of all hydrocephalic children [44]. In the vast majority of these patients, the cause of the hydrocephalus is obvious to the attending surgeon, who has repaired the patient's myelomeningocele. More diagnostic difficulties arise in these patients in the setting of shunt failures and isolated fourth ventricles (discussed below) than in the initial diagnosis of hydrocephalus.

Hydrocephalus is present in 70–80% of patients with the *Dandy-Walker malformation* [38, 62]. However, hydrocephalus is uncommonly present at birth and frequently does not become evident until after infancy. The reason for the delayed appearance of hydrocephalus in Dandy-Walker patients has not been established. It has been suggested that the large posterior fossa cyst makes these patients more susceptible to subarachnoid hemorrhage resulting from minor trauma; the subarachnoid blood may then impede the absorption of CSF, resulting in hydrocephalus [38]. The fact that the location of the block to CSF flow in the Dandy-Walker malformation does not appear consistent [36, 38] is compatible with this theory. Obstruction to CSF flow is usually found at or distal to the fourth ventricle outflow foramina [38, 51]; therefore, the aqueduct is patent (fig. 11) and shunting of the posterior fossa cyst often results in satisfactory decompression of the ventricular system. However, occasionally, an obstruction may be present at the aqueduct, as well. New MR CSF flow studies [1, 46, 61] may be useful in assessing the location(s) of the obstruction(s) and guiding the placement of the initial shunt.

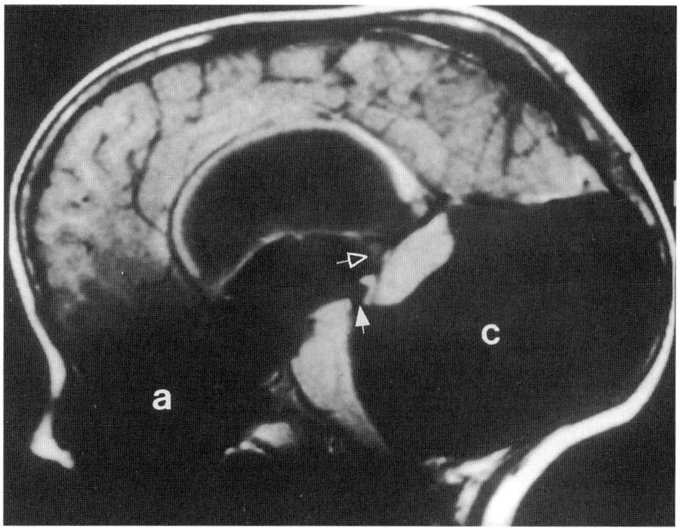

Fig. 11. Dandy-Walker malformation. Sagittal T1-weighted image, somewhat distorted by artifact (a) from metallic dental work. The posterior fossa is expanded by the fourth ventricular-cisterna magna cyst (c). The lateral ventricle, third ventricle, and aqueduct (closed arrow) are markedly dilated, Note the expanded suprapineal recess (open arrow).

It has been shown that, in the absence of associated anomalies, patients with Dandy-Walker malformations can have normal intelligence and lead normal lives if their hydrocephalus is controlled [5, 31, 48]. Examination by MR is of great prognostic significance because MR is more sensitive than other imaging modalities in the detection of areas of damaged or dysgenetic brain [48].

It should be noted that patients with agenesis or hypogenesis of the corpus callosum will frequently have enlarged trigones, occipital horns, and temporal horns of the lateral ventricles, a condition known as colpocephaly (fig. 12). It is important to recognize the normal size and crescentic shape of the frontal horns and bodies of the lateral ventricles in order to identify this condition as a malformation and avoid unnecessary CSF diversion procedures [6].

Isolated (Trapped) Fourth Ventricle

On imaging studies, the isolated fourth ventricle appears as a large rounded or pear-shaped midline cystic structure in the posterior fossa [66]. Sagittal images may show wall of the ventricle bulging superiorly behind the quadrigeminal plate. The lateral and third ventricles are small or only moderately enlarged if the lateral ventriculoperitoneal shunt is functioning. The aqueduct is always narrowed (fig. 13).

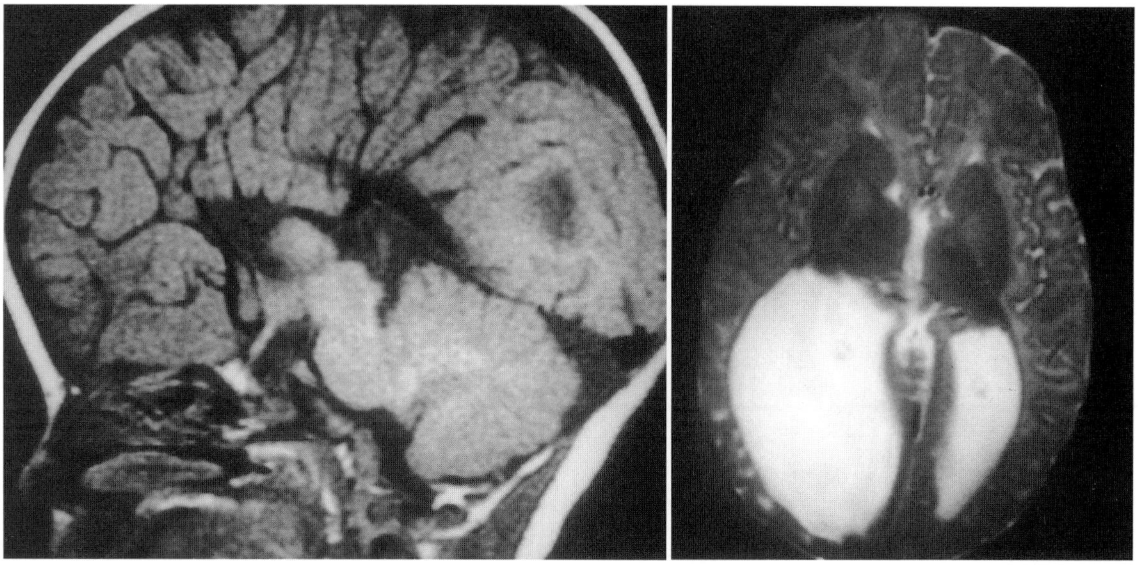

A B

Fig. 12. Agenesis of the corpus callosum with colpocephaly. **A** Saggital T1-weighted image shows the medial hemispheric sulci radiating all the way into the third ventricle without normal cingulate gyrus, cingulate sulcus, and corpus callosum. **B** Axial T2-weighted image shows markedly enlarged occipital horns and trigones with normal-sized frontal horns. This is a developmental anomaly, not hydrocephalus.

Hydrocephalus Secondary to Extraventricular Obstruction of CSF (Communicating Hydrocephalus)

Communicating hydrocephalus represents approximately 30% of all childhood hydrocephalus [29]. Causes include arachnoidal inflammation and scarring from trauma, hemorrhage or infection, blockage by acute hemorrhage or subarachnoid tumor, and increased pressure in the dural venous sinuses. In general, it is not possible to determine the level of the extraventricular obstruction to CSF flow from imaging studies. However, certain features seen on imaging studies can help to differentiate the different causes of the hydrocephalus. For example, hemorrhage often leaves hemosiderin staining of the parenchyma, ependyma, or pia-arachnoid (superficial siderosis). The hemosiderin will appear black on long TR spin-echo images [32, 33] and especially so on gradient echo images [75]. Both meningitis and subarachnoid tumor may result in meningeal enhancement after administration of intravenous contrast [52, 53, 63]. Differentiation of subarachnoid tumor from infection, however, is not possible at this time by radiologic methods.

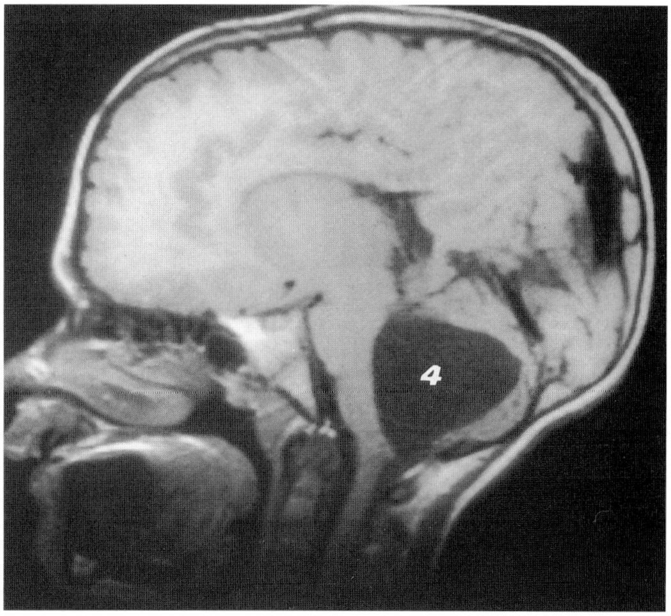

Fig. 13. Isolated third ventricle. Sagittal T1-weighted image shows a very enlarged fourth ventricle (4) despite adequate decompression of the lateral and third ventricles. The brainstem is anteriorly displaced and the cerebellum posteriorly displaced by the enlarged fourth ventricle.

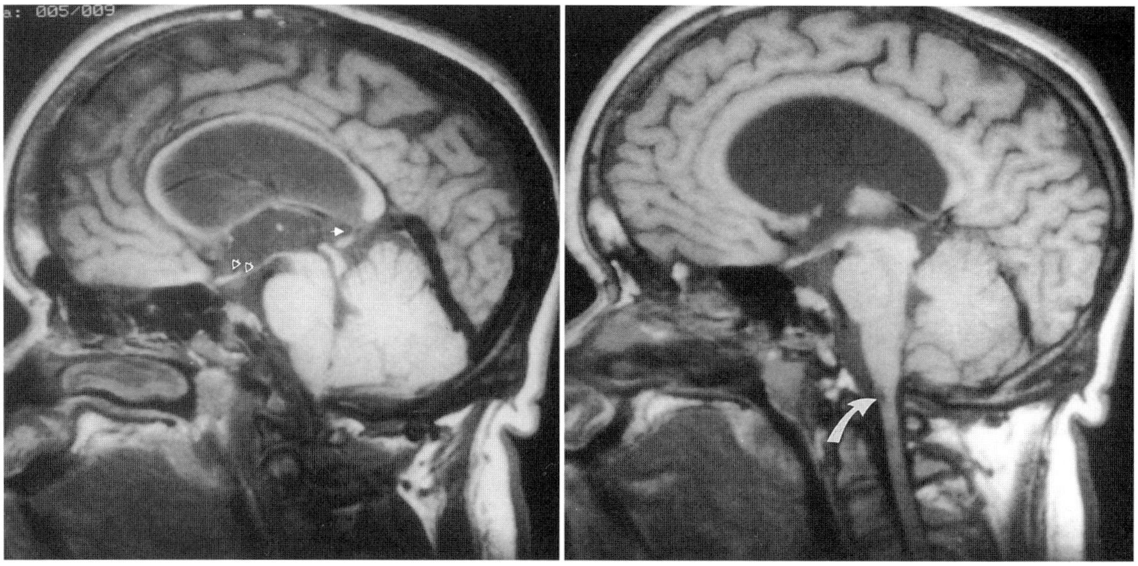

14A 14B

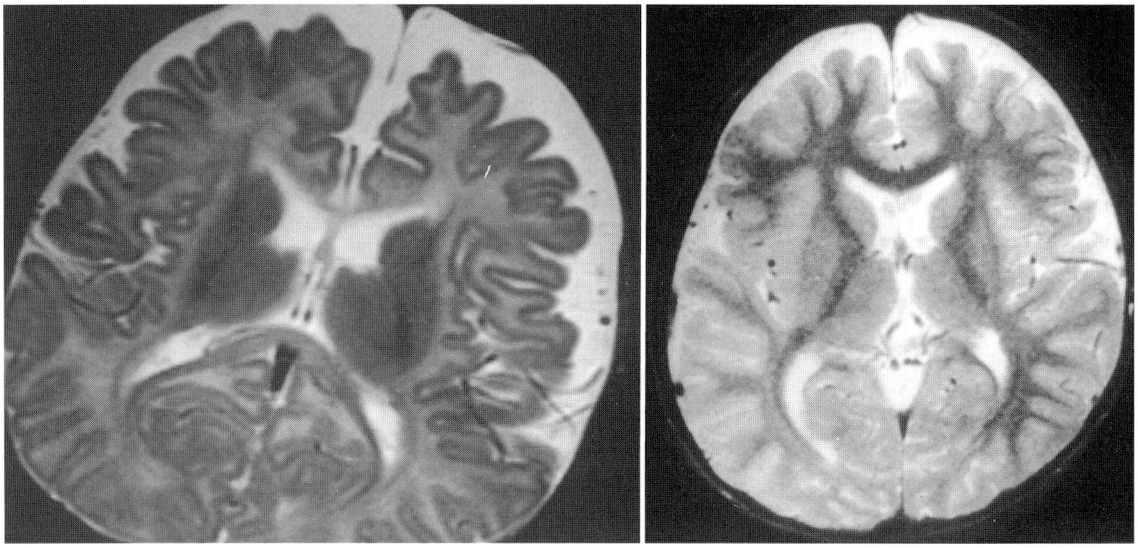

15A 15B

Fig. 14. Achondroplasia. Adjacent sagittal T1-weighted images **(A, B)** show enlarged lateral and third ventricles. Note the dilated anterior (open arrows) and posterior (closed arrow) recesses of the third ventricle. Note also the small clivus and narrow foramen magnum that are characteristic of this disease. Some hypointensity at the cervicomedullary junction (curved arrow) indicates damage from the stenosis at the foramen magnum.

Fig. 15. Benign external hydrocephalus. **A** Axial T2-weighted image obtained at age 6 months shows slightly enlarged ventricles and very large extra-axial (subarachnoid vs. subdural) fluid collections. **B** Follow-up scan at age 18 months shows marked diminution in the size of the fluid collections.

Increased Venous Pressure

Increased intracranial venous pressure may produce either hydrocephalus or pseudotumor cerebri, depending upon the patient's age [64]. Hydrocephalus is more likely if the patient is less than 18 months of age, whereas pseudotumor cerebri is noted if the patient is more than 3 years of age. This difference is thought to result from an expandable calvarium and softer, less myelinated parenchyma in the infant which allows greater ventricular dilatation under high pressure [23, 39, 68, 69]. Once the sutures are fused or the calvarium is artificially prevented from expanding, intracranial hypertension occurs without ventricular enlargement and results in pseudotumor cerebri [23, 69]. It has been postulated that the ventricular enlargement in achondroplasia (fig. 14) results from diminished venous outflow through the hypoplastic skull base [47, 73]. Although MR angiography can show the jugular veins and can measure the velocity of their blood flow as they exit the calvarium through the jugular foramina, the measurement of pressure differentials does not seem possible at this time.

Benign Enlargement of the Subarachnoid Spaces in Infants

The CT and MR pattern of enlarged CSF spaces and normal to slightly increased ventricular size (fig. 15) in infants with macrocephaly or rapid head growth is fairly common [7, 11, 12, 59]. This phenomenon has been variously called benign extra-axial collections of infancy, external hydrocephalus, extraventricular obstructive hydrocephalus, benign subdural effusion of infancy, benign macrocephaly of infancy, and benign enlargement of the subarachnoid spaces. The significance of this finding and, indeed, the actual location of these fluid collections (subarachnoid versus subdural) has been a subject of much debate [7, 12, 59].

In the absence of underlying brain anomalies, these children tend to develop normally [59]. Their head circumference tends to be in the high normal range at birth, but increases rapidly during the first few months of life; it is generally well above the 95th percentile at the time of presentation (usually between the ages of 2 and 7 months). It is important to recognize that, in the absence of developmental delay or signs or symptoms of increased intracranial pressure, this rapid head growth may not represent hydrocephalus or the presence of subdural hematomas. In fact, when followed without intervention, these infants' head growth tends to stabilize along a curve parallel to the 95th percentile by the age of 18 months; both the size of the extra-axial spaces and the head circumference often return to normal after the 2nd birthday [12]. Cisternography has demonstrated slow flow over the cerebral convexities in these patients [11]; the enlarged subarachnoid spaces may therefore result from delayed maturation of the arachnoid villi.

Enlarged subarachnoid spaces can be caused by a number of factors, including ACTH and corticosteroid therapy [34, 41] and cancer chemotherapy, in addition to the mechanisms discussed previously in this manuscript. Imaging studies are often not helpful in the distinction of benign macrocephaly of infancy from hydrocephalus or, for that matter, from atrophy. As discussed earlier, scrutiny of the anterior and posterior recesses of the third ventricle and the temporal horns may be helpful in the differentiation from hydrocephalus (fig. 3). Symmetry of the extra-axial collections is an important finding, especially on CT; asymmetry is unusual in benign macrocephaly and may indicate the presence of traumatic subdural hematomas [54]. In the absence of clinical signs of symptoms, cisternography is probably not indicated.

The authors have encountered several patients with clinical courses strongly suggestive of benign macrocephaly of infancy who have had bloody subdural collections detected on MR scans (fig. 16). Extensive investigations have revealed no evidence of significant trauma. It is postulated that the large CSF spaces in these patients may make them more susceptible to subdural hematoma formation secondary to rather mild trauma, similar to the condition encountered in patients with middle cranial fossa arachnoid cysts [30, 57].

Treatment of Hydrocephalus and the Resulting Complications

Shunt Malfunction

On imaging studies, shunt malfunction is usually manifested by increasing ventricular size. However, some patients have considerable scarring in and around the ventricular walls causing a decreased compliance of the brain; such patients may show no enlargement or minimal enlargement of the ventricular system in the presence of shunt malfunction [24, 60]. The most common malfunction is that of occlusion of the ventricular catheter by choroid plexus or glial tissue that grows into the lumen of the catheter. This diagnosis can oly be inferred from static imaging studies and plain x-rays, which will show enlarging lateral ventricles in spite of a well-placed ventriculostomy tube and intact connections of the shunt system. Disconnection can occur at any point within the system; it most commonly occurs where the various components are joined. This diagnosis can usually be made by plain film examination of the entire shunt system [55]. Although the site of shunt malfunction (ventricular portion vs. peritoneal portion) can generally be determined clinically, it is occasionally necessary to determine the site of shunt obstruction using positive contrast plain film radiography or radionuclide studies [25, 35, 40, 74]. Shuntograms are of value when symptoms of shunt malfunction are vague and clinical testing of shunt function is equivo-

A B

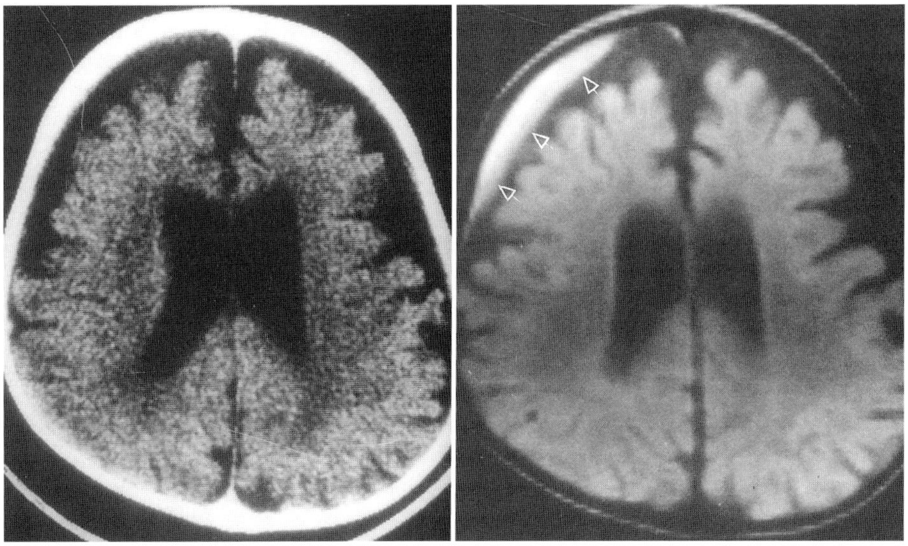

Fig. 16. Subdural hematoma associated with benign external hydrocephalus. **A** Axial CT scan at age 5 months shows large ventricles and large amount of extra-axial fluid in this patient with macrocephaly but normal development and normal neurological exam, compatible with benign external hydrocephalus. **B** Axial MR scan obtained as a routine follow-up shows a right frontal subdural hematoma (arrows).

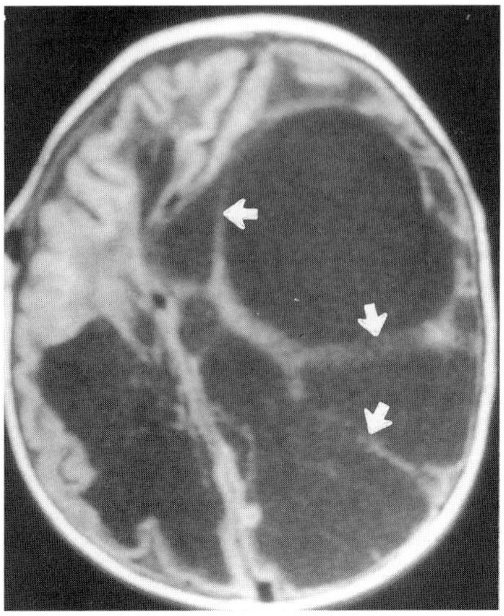

Fig. 17. Sequelae of ventriculitis. Axial T1-weighted MR scan shows multiple loculations within and external to the lateral ventricles, separated by thin septa (arrows).

cal. They show qualitatively, and in some radionuclide studies quantitatively [35, 40], the flow of CSF through the shunt system.

Advances in the analysis of CSF flow have recently allowed flow to be detected in ventricular catheters and in connecting tubing [13, 49]. Parameters can be set to detect flow that is more rapid than a certain minimum velocity. If flow is seen within the shunt tubing, one may be confident that a certain level of flow is present in that portion of the shunt system. Unfortunately, the inconsistent nature of CSF production makes a negative study (no flow) less valuable; a negative study does not necessarily mean that the shunt system has failed [13]. A more conventional shuntogram is then required

Infection

The risk of infection resulting from ventricular shunting has decreased steadily over the years and is now generally between 1 and 5% [29]. The only aspect of shunt infection that is visualized on imaging studies is that of ventriculitis, which is seen on contrast-enhanced imaging studies as enlarged lateral ventricles with an irregular, enhancing ventricular wall. Septations can sometimes be seen within the ventricles, most easily detected by ultrasonography [2]. The three-dimensional imaging capability of MR is extremely helpful in identifying and localizing each loculation within the ventricular system. Occasionally, after severe ventriculitis, the multiple loculations can cause distortion of the brain, resulting in a confusing image (fig. 17).

Subdural Hematomas

Other complications resulting from ventriculoperitoneal shunting are much less common. Complications within the abdomen include ascites, pseudocyst formation, perforation of a viscus or of the abdominal wall, and intestinal obstruction [16, 35]. Significant subdural hematomas (fig. 18) are unusual after shunting. These subdural fluid collections are usually seen in children over 3 years of age after overly vigorous drainage of markedly enlarged ventricles [60]. The use of high pressure valves in the shunting of these patients has reduced the incidence of significant subdural hematomas. Small subdural hematomas are often seen on MR scans of patients who have recently been shunted because of its sensitivity to even very small subdural fluid collections (fig. 19). These small hematomas are almost never of clinical significance.

Using contrast-enhanced MR or CT, chronic subdural hematomas can be distinguished from postshunt meningeal fibrosis (meningeal callus, [26]), in which a thick collagenous scar develops in the subdural space, presumably as a reaction to chronic subdural hematoma [17, 19, 26].

A B

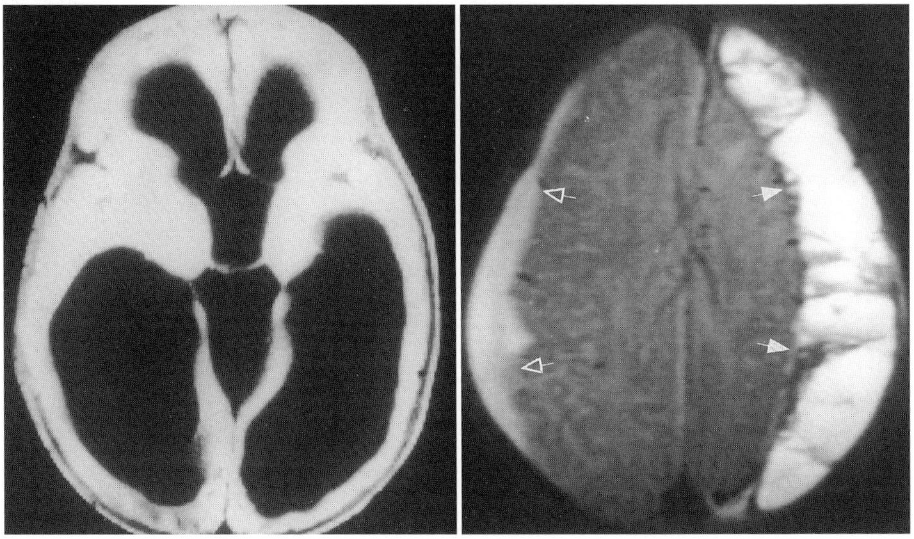

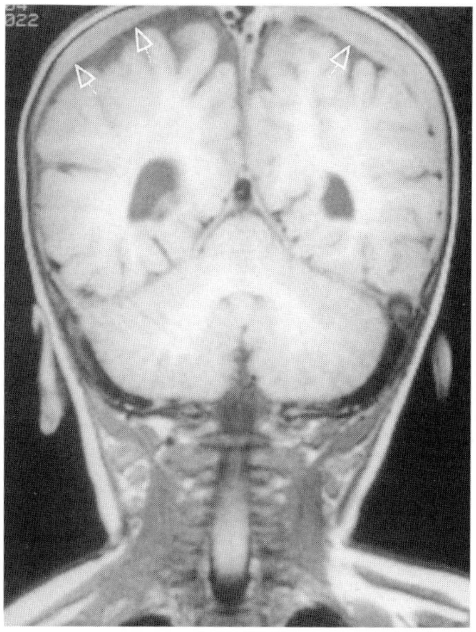

Fig. 18. Large subdural hematoma. **A** Axial T1-weighted image before shunting shows severe hydrocephalus. **B** Axial T2-weighted image after shunting shows a small, chronic subdural hematoma (open arrows) on the right and a larger subacute subdural hematoma (closed arrows) on the left. The subdural on the left was bright on both T1- and T2-weighted images, indicating the presence of methemoglobin. The smaller right subdural collection was dark on T1-weighted images, indicating resorption of all methemoglobin and, hence, chronicity [from 2, with permission].

Fig. 19. Bilateral small, asymptomatic subdural hematomas after ventriculoperitoneal shunting. Arrows mark the inner layer of the dura, separating the hypointense fluid in the subarachnoid space from the more hyperintense fluid in the subdural space.

A B C

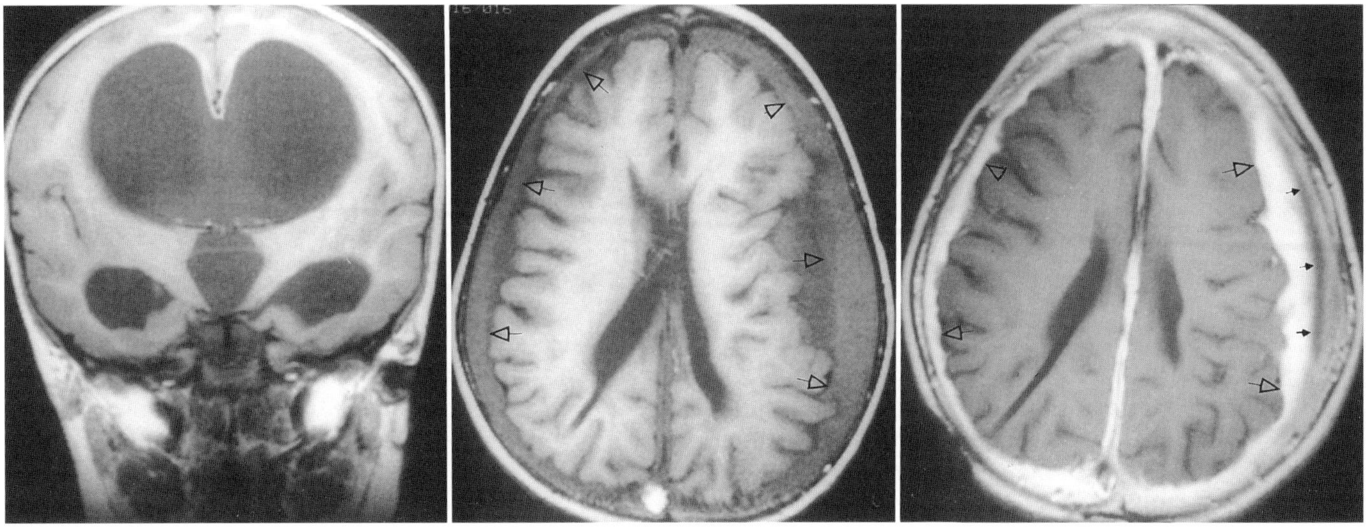

Fig. 20. Postshunt meningeal fibrosis. **A** Prior to shunting, the patient has marked hydrocephalus, with dilated, rounded lateral ventricular bodies, third ventricle, and temporal horns. **B** Follow-up axial T1-weighted noncontrast scan shows a low-to-intermediate intensity substance (arrows) in the subdural spaces bilaterally. **C** Following contrast administration, most of the subdural material enhances markedly (large open arrows). A small amount of the subdural material (small closed arrows) does not enhance and may represent residual fluid or nonvascular fibrous tissue.

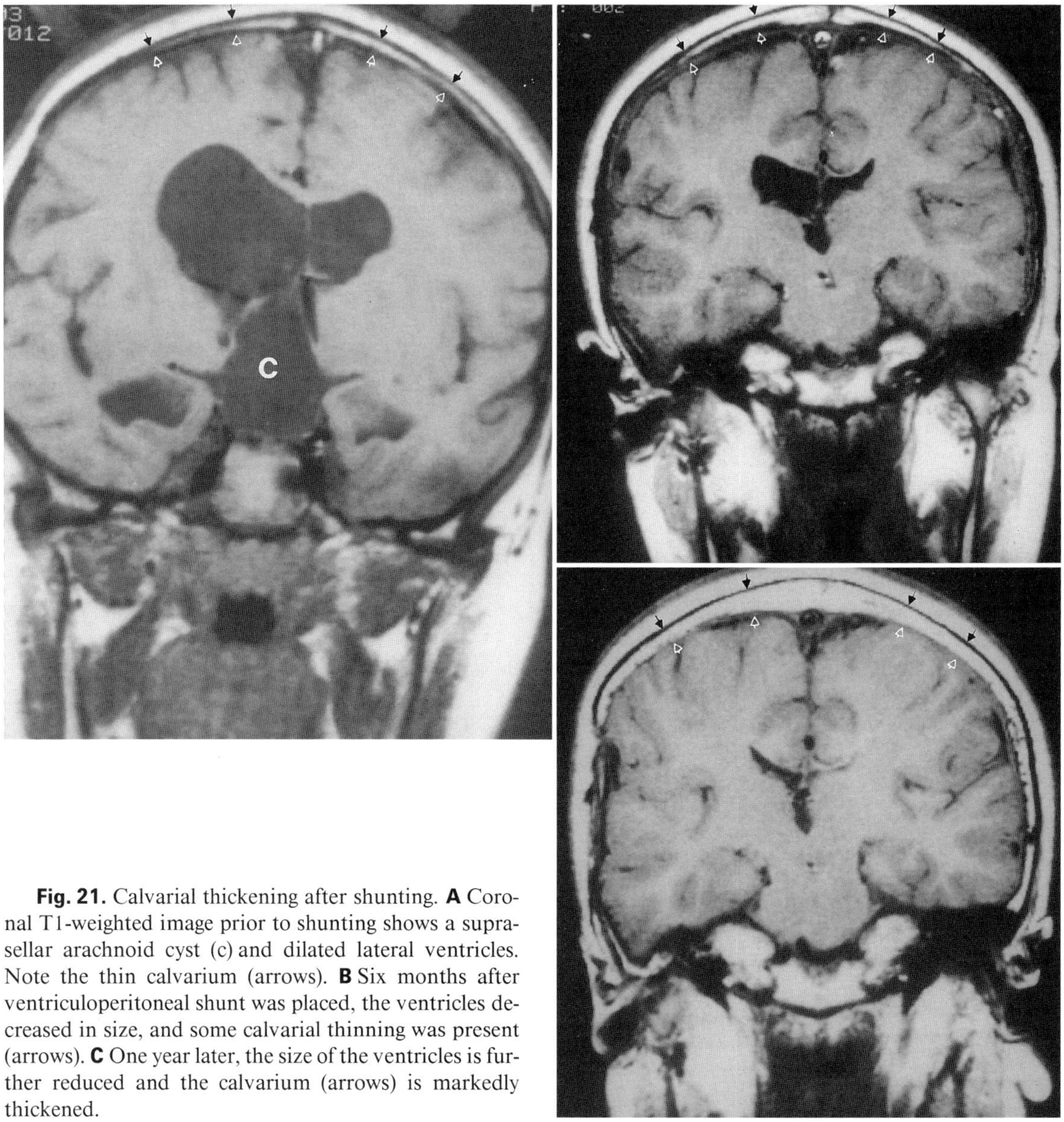

A B C

Fig. 21. Calvarial thickening after shunting. **A** Coronal T1-weighted image prior to shunting shows a suprasellar arachnoid cyst (c) and dilated lateral ventricles. Note the thin calvarium (arrows). **B** Six months after ventriculoperitoneal shunt was placed, the ventricles decreased in size, and some calvarial thinning was present (arrows). **C** One year later, the size of the ventricles is further reduced and the calvarium (arrows) is markedly thickened.

Whereas chronic subdural hematomas will not enhance after administration of contrast, meningeal fibrosis enhances dramatically (fig. 20), presumably as a result of vascular granulation tissue intermixed with the collagen bundles in the subdural space [17].

Slit Ventricle Syndrome

Shunted hydrocephalic patients may become symptomatic from shunt failure in the absence of ventricular enlargement as detected by CT or MR. This has been called the 'slit ventricle syndrome' [21, 22, 24]. Some debate exists as to what constellation of clinical and/or pathological findings define this syndrome [24, 67]. Most likely, the syndrome is the result of diminished brain compliance, diminished ability to compensate for the normal variations in intracranial pressure (probably secondary to a decreased intracranial volume of CSF), and, possibly, intermittent or partial shunt obstruction [24, 60]. It is important to realize that the presence of very small ventricles after placement of a ventriculoperitoneal

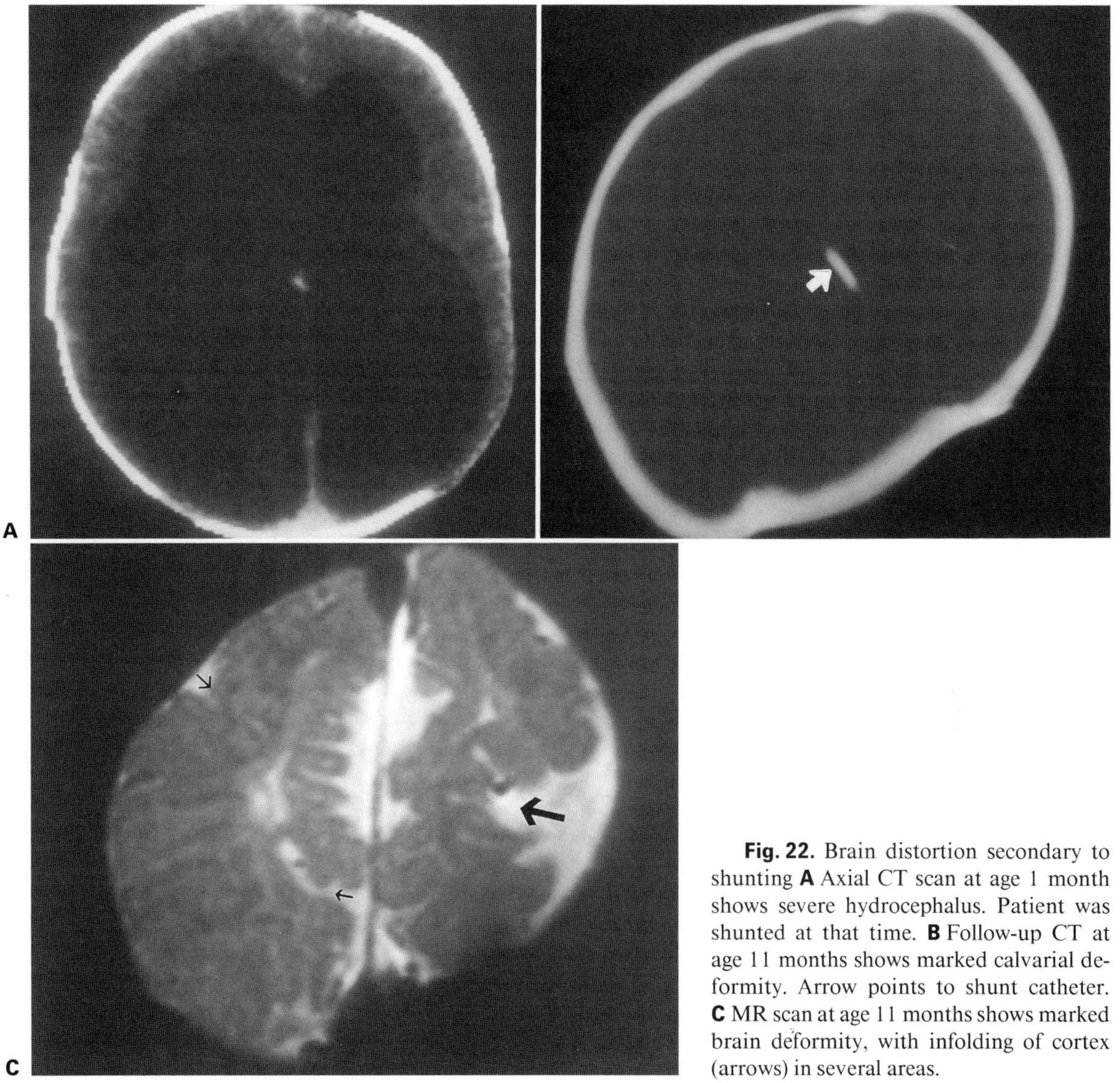

Fig. 22. Brain distortion secondary to shunting **A** Axial CT scan at age 1 month shows severe hydrocephalus. Patient was shunted at that time. **B** Follow-up CT at age 11 months shows marked calvarial deformity. Arrow points to shunt catheter. **C** MR scan at age 11 months shows marked brain deformity, with infolding of cortex (arrows) in several areas.

shunt is not diagnostic of, or even suggestive of, the slit ventricle syndrome. Small ventricles are the desired result of many surgeons after ventriculoperitoneal shunting and, even when extremely small, their only implication in the vast majority of patients is that the shunt is functioning.

One finding on imaging studies that may help in the determination of which patients have the slit ventricle syndrome is that of calvarial thickening (fig. 21). Such thickening may be associated with premature synostosis of the cranial sutures and a resultant diminished reservoir of CSF to buffer the normal variations in intracranial pressure [24].

Other Complications

Infants who are shunted for severe hydrocephalus sometimes end up with premature closure of their calvarial sutures, i.e., premature craniosynostosis. At times, the sutures can fuse in a bizarre configuration (fig. 22). More commonly, the patients develop chronic subdural hematomas that eventually become fibrotic [17] and the skull thickens (fig. 21).

Very rarely patients may develop a granulomatous reaction adjacent to the shunt tube either within or near the ventricle [14]. These granulomatous lesions appear as irregular, contrast-enhancing masses along the course of the shunt tube. Calcification may be noted within the mass.

One final appearance of shunt malfunction should be mentioned. Rarely, when the ventricular end of the shunt becomes partially occluded, CSF may track along this shunt and enter the interstices of the centrum semiovale. On these occasions, the CT and MR appearance is that of edema (low density in the white matter on CT, prolonged T1 and T2 relaxation time in the white matter on MR) in the area around the shunt [2]. Eventually, an actual cyst may form in the white matter surrounding the ventriuclar catheter. It should be recognized that the presence of edema in these patients is not the result of infection or tumor but is a sign of shunt malfunction. The edema and cyst will resolve after shunt revision.

References

1 Atlas S, Mark A, Fram E: Aqueductal stenosis: Evaluation with gradient echo rapid MR imaging. Radiology 1988;169:449–453.

2 Barkovich A: Hydrocephalus; in Barkovich A (ed): Pediatric Neuroimaging. New York, Raven Press, 1990, pp 205–226.

3 Barkovich A, Edwards M: Brain tumors of childhood; in Barkovich A (ed): Pediatric Neuroimaging. New York, Raven Press, 1990, pp 149–203.

4 Barkovich A, Newton T: Aqueductal stenosis: Evidence of a broad spectrum of tectal distortion. AJNR 1989;10:471–475.

5 Barkovich AJ, Kjos BO, Norman D, Edwards MSB: Revised classification of posterior fossa cysts and cyst-like malformations based on results of multiplanar MR imaging. AJNR 1989; 10:977–988.

6 Barkovich AJ, Norman D: Anomalies of the corpus callosum: Correlation with further anomalies of the brain. AJNR 1988;9:493–501.

7 Barlow C: CSF dynamics in hydrocephalus – With special attention to external hydrocephalus. Brain Dev 1984;6:119–127.

8 Borit A, Sidman RL: New mutant mouse with communicating hydrocephalus and secondary aqueductal stenosis. Acta Neuropathol 1972; 21:316–331.

9 Bradley W Jr, Kortman K, Burgoyne B, Eng D: Flowing cerebrospinal fluid in normal and hydrocephalic states. Appearance on MR images. Radiology 1986;159:611–616.

10 Bradley W Jr, Whittemore A, Kortman K, Watanabe A, Homyak M, Teresi L, Davis S: Marked cerebrospinal fluid void: Indicator of successful shunt in patients with suspected normal-pressure hydrocephalus. Radiology 1991; 178:459–466.

11 Briner S, Bodensteiner J: Benign subdural collection of infancy. Pediatrics 1980;67:802–804.

12 Carolan PL, McLaurin RL, Robin RB, Tobin JA, Egelhoff JC: Benign extra-axial collections of infancy. Pediatr Neurosci 1986;12:140–144.

13 Castillo M, Hudgins P, Malko J, Burrow B, Hoffman J Jr: Flow-sensitive MR imaging of ventriculoperitoneal shunts: In vitro findings, clinical applications, and pitfalls. AJNR 1991; 12:667–672.

14 Citrin C, Hammock M: Computed tomographic representation of granulomatous reaction from intraventricular shunt. Comput Tomogr 1979;3:177–180.

15 Coates T, Hinshaw D Jr, Peckman N, et al: Pediatric choroid plexus neoplasms: MR, CT, and pathologic correlations. Radiology 1989; 173:81–88.

16 Davidson RI: Peritoneal bypass in the treatment of hydrocephalus: Historical review of abdominal complications. J Neurol Neurosurg Psychiatry 1976;39:640–648.

17 Destian S, Heier L, Zimmerman R, et al: Differentiation between meningeal fibrosis and chronic subdural hematoma after ventricular shunting: Value of enhanced CT and MR scans. AJNR 1989;10:1021–1026.

18 El Gammal T, Allen M Jr, Brooks B, Mark E: MR evaluation of hydrocephalus. AJNR 1987; 8:591–597.

19 Emery J: Intracranial effects of long-standing decompression of the brain in children with hydrocephalus and meningomyelocele. Dev Med Child Neurol 1965;7:302–309.

20 Enzmann D, Pelc N: Normal flow patterns of intracranial and spinal cerebrospinal fluid defined with phase-contrast cine MR imaging. Radiology 1991;178:467–474.

21 Epstein F, Fleisher A, Hochwald G, Ransohoff J: Subtemporal craniectomy for recurrent shunt obstruction secondary to small ventricles. J Neurosurg 1974;41:29–31.

22 Epstein F, Hochwald G, Wald A, Ransohoff J: Avoidance of shunt dependency in hydrocephalus. Dev Med Child Neurol 1975;17:71–77.

23 Epstein F, Hochwald GM, Ransohoff J: Neonatal hydrocephalus treated by compressive head wrapping. Lancet 1973;i:634.

24 Epstein F, Lapras C, Wisoff JH: 'Slit ventricle syndrome': Etiology and treatment. Pediatr Neurosci 1988;14:5–10.

25 Evans RC, Thomas MD, Williams LA: Shunt blockage in hydrocephalic children. The use of the valvogram. Clin Radiol 1976;27:489.

26 Falhauer KP: Overdrainage phenomena in shunt treated hydrocepalus. Acta Neurochir (Wien) 1978;45:89–101.

27 Fitz C: Neoplastic diseases; In Gonzales C, Grossman C, Masdeu J (eds): Head and Spine Imaging. New York, Wiley 1985, pp 385–410.

28 Fitz CR, Harwood-Nash DC: Computed tomography of hydrocephalus. Comput Tomogr 1978;2:91–108.

29 Gabriel R, McComb J: Malformations of the central nervous system, in Menkes J (ed): Textbook of Child Neurology. Philadelphia, Lea & Febiger, 1985, pp 234–253.

30 Galassi E, Tognetti F, Gaist G, et al: CT scan and metrizamide cisternography in arachnoid cysts of the middle cranial fossa: Classification and pathophysiological aspects. Surg Neurol 1982;17:363–369.

31 Golden JA, Rorke LB, Bruce DA: Dandy-Walker syndrome and associated anomalies. Pediatr Neurosci. 1987;13:38–44.

32 Gomori J, Grossman R, Goldberg H, et al: High field spin echo MR imaging of superficial and subependymal siderosis secondary to neonatal intraventricular hemorrhage. Neuroradiology 1987;29:339.

33 Gomori J, Grossman R, Goldberg H, Zimmerman R, Bilaniuk L: Intracranial hematomas: Imaging by high field MR. Radiology 1985; 157:87.

34 Gordon N: Apparent cerebral atrophy in patients on treatment with steroids. Dev Med Child Neurol 1980;22:502–506.

35 Guertin S: Cerebrospinal fluid shunts. Evaluation, complications, and crisis management. Pediatr Clin North Am 1987;34:203–217.

36 Hart M, Malamud N, Ellis W: The Dandy-Walker syndrome. A clinicopathological study based on 28 cases. Neurology 1972;22:771–780.

37 Heinz ER, Ward A, Drayer BP, DuBois PJ: Distinction between obstructive and atrophic dilatation of ventricles in children. J Comput Assist Tomogr 1980;4:320–325.

38 Hirsch J, Pierre-Kahn A, Renier D, Sainte-Rose C, Hoppe-Hirsch E: The Dandy-Walker malformation: A review of 40 cases. J Neurosurg 1984;61:515–522.

39 Hochwald G, Epstein F, Malhan C, et al: The role of skull and dural in experimental feline hydrocephalus. Dev Med Child Neurol 1972; 14(suppl 27):65–69.

40 Howman-Giles R, McLaughlin A, Johnston I, Whittle I: A radionuclide method of evaluating shunt function and CSF circulation in hydrocephalus. Technical note. J Neurosurg 1984; 61:604–605.

41 Ito M, Takao P, Okumo T, Mikawa H: Sequential CT studies of 24 children with infantile spasms on ACTH therapy. Dev Med Child Neurol 1983;25:475–480.

42 Kim C, Bennett D, Roberts T: Primary amenorrhea secondary to noncommunicating hydrocephalus. Neurology 1969;19:533–537.

43 Kleinman P, Zito J, Davidson R, Raptopoulos V: The subarachnoid spaces in children: Normal variations in size. Radiology 1983;147:455–457.

44 Laurence K: The pathology of hydrocephalus. Ann R Coll Surg 1959;24:388.

45 LeMay M, Hochberg F: Ventricular differences between hydrostatic hydrocephalus and hydrocephalus ex vacuo by computed tomography. Neuroradiology 1979;17:191–195.

46 Levy L, Di Chiro G: MR phase imaging and cerebrospinal fluid flow in the head and spine. Neuroradiology 1990;32:399–406.

47 Lundar T, Bakke S, Nornes H: Hydrocephalus in an achondroplastic child treated by venous decompression at the jugular foramen. Case report. J Neurosurg 1990;73:138–140.

48 Maria B, Zinreich S, Carson B, Rosenbaum A, Freeman J: Dandy-Walker syndrome revisited. Pediatr Neurosurg 1987;13:45–51.

49 Martin A, Drake J, Lemaire C, Henkelman R: Cerebrospinal fluid shunts. Flow measurements with MR imaging. Radiology 1989;173:243–247.

50 Martin N, Pierot L, Sterkers O, Mompoint D, Nahum H: Primary choroid plexus papilloma of the cerebellopontine angle: MR imaging. Neuroradiology 1990;31:541–543.

51 Masdeu J, Dobben G, Azar-Kia B: Dandy-Walker syndrome studied by computed tomography and pneumoencephalography. Radiology 1983;147:109–114.

52 Mathews V, Kuharit M, Edwards M, D'Amour P, Azzarelli B, Dreesen R: Gadolinium enhanced MR imaging of experimental bacterial meningitis: Evaluation and comparison with CT. AJNR 1988;9:1045–1050.

53 Matthews V, Broome D, Smith R, Bognanno J, Einhorn L, Edwards M: Neuroimaging of disseminated germ cell tumors. AJNR 1990;11:319–324.

54 Maytal J, Alvarez L, Elkin C, Shinnar S: External hydrocephalus: Radiologic spectrum and differentiation from cerebral atrophy. AJNR 1987;8:271–278.

55 Naidich T, Gado M: Hydrocephalus; In Newton T, Potts D (eds): Ventricles and Cisterns. St. Louis, Mosby, 1978 chap 107.

56 Naidich T, McLone D, Hahn Y, Hanaway J: Atrial diverticula in severe hydrocephalus. AJNR 1982;3:257–266.

57 Naidich T, McLone D, Radkowski M: Intracranial arachnoid cysts. Pediatr Neurosci 1986;12:112–122.

58 Naidich T, Zimmerman R: Primary brain tumors in children. Semin Roentgenol 1984;19:100–114.

59 Nickel R, Gallenstein J: Developmental prognosis for infants with benign enlargement of the subarachnoid spaces. Dev Med Child Neurol 1987;29:181–186.

60 Oi S, Matsumoto S: Infantile hydrocephalus and the slit ventricle syndrome in early infancy. Childs Nerv Syst 1987;3:145–150.

61 Quencer R, Post M, Hinks R: Cine MR in the evaluation of normal and abnormal CSF flow: Intracranial and intraspinal studies. Neuroradiology 1990;32:371–391.

62 Raimondi A, Sato K, Shimoji T: The Dandy-Walker syndrome. Basel, Karger, 1984.

63 Rippe D, Boyko O, Friedman H, et al: Gd-DTPA-enhanced MR imaging of leptomeningeal spread of primary intracranial CNS tumors in children. AJNR 1990;11:329–332.

64 Rosman N, Shands K: Hydrocephalus caused by increased intracranial venous pressure: A clinicopathological study. Ann Neurol 1978;3:445–450.

65 Russell D: Observations on the pathology of hydrocephalus. Medical Research Council Special Reports Series. London, HMSO 1949, No 265, pp. 1–138.

66 Scotti G, Musgrave M, Fitz C, Harwood-Nash D: The isolated fourth ventricle in children: CT and clinical review of 16 cases. Am J Roentgenol 1980;135:1233–1238.

67 Serlo W, Heikkinen E, Saukkonen A-L, Wendt L: Classification and management of the slit ventricle syndrome. Child Nerv Syst 1985;1:194–199.

68 Shapiro K, Fried A, Maramou A: Biomechanical and hydrodynamic characterization of the hydrocephalic infant. J Neurosurg 1985;63:69–75.

69 Shapiro K, Fried A, Takei F, Kohn I: Effect of the skull and dura on neural axis pressure-volume relationships and CSF hydrodynamics. J Neurosurg 1985;63:76–81.

70 Sherman J, Citrin C: Magnetic resonance of normal CSF flow. AJNR 1986;7:3–6.

71 Sherman J, Citrin C, Gangarosa R, Bowen B: The MR appearance of CSF flow in patients with ventriculomegaly. AJNR 1986;7:1025–1031.

72 Sjaastad O, Skalpe I, Engeset A: The width of the temporal horn and the differential diagnosis between pressure hydrocephalus and hydrocephalus ex vacuo. Neurology 1969;19:1087–1093.

73 Steinbok P, Hall J, Flodmark O: Hydrocephalus in achondroplasia: The possible role of intracranial venous hypertension. J Neurosurg 1989;71:42–48.

74 Sweeney L, Thomas P: Contrast examination of cerebrospinal fluid malfunction in infancy and childhood. Pediatr Radiol 1987;17:177–183.

75 Unger E, Cohen M, Brown T: Gradient echo imaging of hermorrhage at 1.5T. Magn Res Imag 1989;7:163–167.

76 Williams B: Is aqueductal stenosis the result of hydrocephalus? Brain 1973;96:399–412.

Pediatr Neurosurg 1992;18:84–91

Diane S. Babcock
Lori L. Barr
Kerry R. Crone

Departments of Radiology, Pediatrics, and Neurosurgery, Children's Hospital Medical Center, and University of Cincinnati, College of Medicine, Cincinnati, Ohio, USA

Intraoperative Uses of Ultrasound in the Pediatric Neurosurgical Patient

Key Words
Brain, ultrasound studies
Brain, neoplasms, ultrasound studies
Cerebral blood vessels, ultrasound guidance
Ultrasound in infants and children

Abstract
Ultrasound imaging has become a common method for intraoperative evaluation of the central nervous system. Real-time monitoring aids in guidance for aspiration of fluid collections and placement of catheters as well as the localization and evaluation of masses, and confirmation of their complete removal. Color Doppler is useful in the evaluation of blood flow in arteriovenous malformations, aneurysms, and neoplasms. Consultation among the ultrasound staff, neuroradiologists, and neurosurgeons before the operative procedure maximizes the usefulness of ultrasound, thus aiding in the success of surgery.

Introduction

Ultrasound equipment can be readily taken to the operating room and used to assist the neurosurgeon in a variety of procedures. Common indications for intraoperative ultrasonography include localization of nonpalpable masses, guidance for aspiration of cysts and other fluid collections, guidance for placement of catheters and ventriculoperitoneal shunts, mass evaluation and confirmation of complete removal [1–4]. Color Doppler imaging has been useful in evaluation of arteriovenous malformations, aneurysms, and neoplasms [5–8]. Our prior experience in children has demonstrated the utility of intraoperative sonography in various clinical situations and pathologic conditions [9].

Technique

The intraoperative procedure is simplified if the radiologist reviews the preoperative imaging studies, familiarizes him/herself with the anatomy and pathology, and consults the neuroradiologist or other appropriate subspecialties concerning the findings demonstrated. The case is then discussed with the neurosurgeon/interventionalist to determine the purpose of intraoperative scanning as well as to discuss the type of transducers to be used. The size of the transducer face and the size and position of the acoustic window (anterior fontanelle, burr hole, or operative defect) can then be discussed and planned with the neurosurgeon.

A variety of ultrasound equipment has been utilized during the procedures. Images may be printed on hard copy, a color printer, or recorded on video tape for subsequent photography and review. Two types of transducers are found to be useful: a phased sector of 3.0- to 7.0-MHz frequency with a small aperture width and a linear array of 5.0- or 7.0-MHz frequency and an aperture width of 40 mm. The sector transducer is particularly useful when scanning through a small acoustical window such as a burr hole or fontanelle. The linear array transducer, while larger, has the advantage of better near-field resolution. A transducer equipped with both color and duplex Doppler is useful for evaluation of intracranial blood flow.

Diane S. Babcock, MD
Department of Radiology
Children's Hospital Medical Center
Elland and Bethesda Avenues
Cincinnati, OH 45229-2899 (USA)

1016–2291/92/0182–0084
$2.75/0

Prior to going to the operating room the case is reviewed with the technologist who will be assisting the radiologist and manipulating the settings on the ultrasound machine. Transducers and accessories to be used are selected and stored on the machine and extraneous equipment is removed. The machine should be equipped with at least 2 transducer covers. An extra one is useful in case of contamination or if a second transducer is utilized during the procedure. At least 3 sterile gel packets, several video cassettes, a video tape, and disinfectant wipes should be available. The ultrasound equipment is wiped with disinfectant before leaving the ultrasound laboratory and the transducer is cleaned again outside of the operating room. The operating room should be evaluated ahead of time for the optimal power source for the ultrasound machine and optimal position for viewing the screen. Other equipment in the operating room can cause electrical interference and affect the ultrasound image, especially the electrocautery device. When planning a neurosurgical operating room a separate electrical line for the ultrasound machine should be considered.

Optimally the ultrasound machine should be positioned in the operating room prior to the beginning of the case. Other equipment to be used by the neurosurgeon such as laser equipment, microscope and ventriculoscope may determine the placement of the machine relative to the patient. The radiologist and technologist don the operating room apparel for machine positioning. If a preliminary scrub is performed at ths time, the response time when they are needed is shortened. It may help for the radiologist to visit the operating room during anesthesia induction of the patient to visualize the head position prior to draping. The radiologist is then free to pursue other responsibilities until the time he or she is needed in the operating room. The operating room nurse is given instructions to call the ultrasound team approximately 15 min prior to the time they are needed. This allows the radiologist time to get to the operating room and perform the necessary handscrub, gowning and gloving without increasing anesthesia time.

The transducer and cord are covered with a sterile sheath by the gloved and gowned radiologist (fig. 1). The optimal transducer cover fits a variety of transducers and is flexible enough that it does not damage sensitive neural tissue. We currently use Civco Surgicover 914623 (Cone Instruments, Solon, Ohio). This transducer cover is accordioned into a plastic holder for easy manipulation. Sterile coupling gel is placed into the end of the cover. The technologist holds the transducer as the radiologist extends the cover over the transducer and cord (fig. 1a).

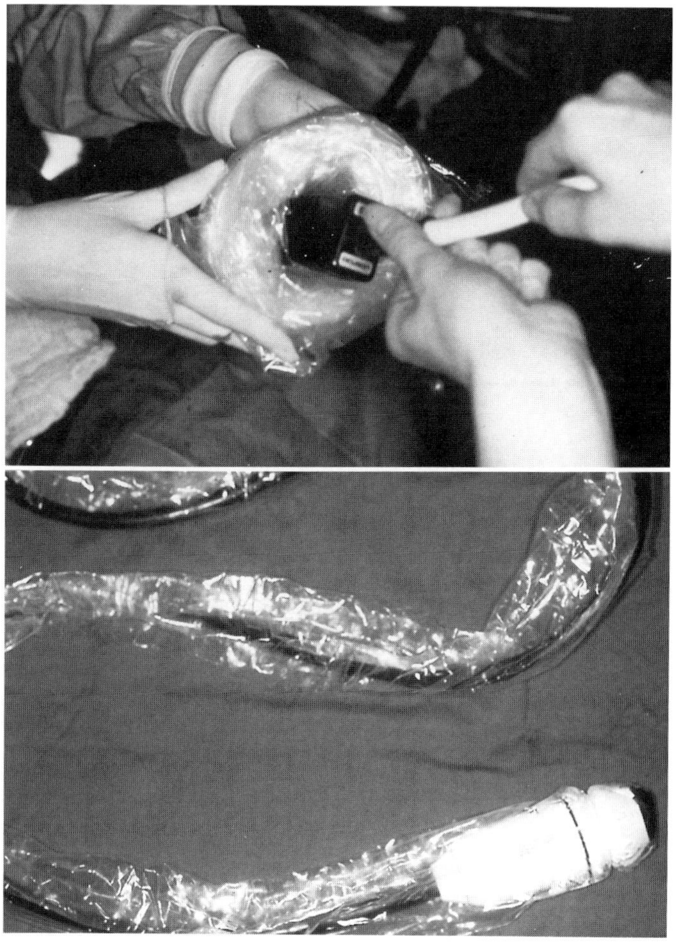

a

b

Fig. 1. Transducer preparation. The transducer and cord are covered with a sterile sheath by the gloved and gowned radiologist. **a** After placing sterile coupling gel in the end of the cover the technologist holds the transducer as the radiologist extends the cover over the transducer and cord. **b** Sheathed transducer.

Sterile rubber bands are then used to secure a bubble-free gel interface over the transducer. Using this technique the sterility of the radiologist is easily maintained while draping the transducer.

We have had only a few complications related to transducer covers (3/150 cases), none of which have occurred since switching to the aforementioned cover. The plastic transducer cover may tear if it comes in contact with a sharp structure such as the cut edge of the bony craniotomy defect, especially if the bone flap is small. Transducer covers made of stiffer plastic can damage underlying neural tissue.

While scanning the head it is helpful to have a stool to sit on to place the radiologist at the level of the patient. It is also helpful to have a holder or other structure for stabi-

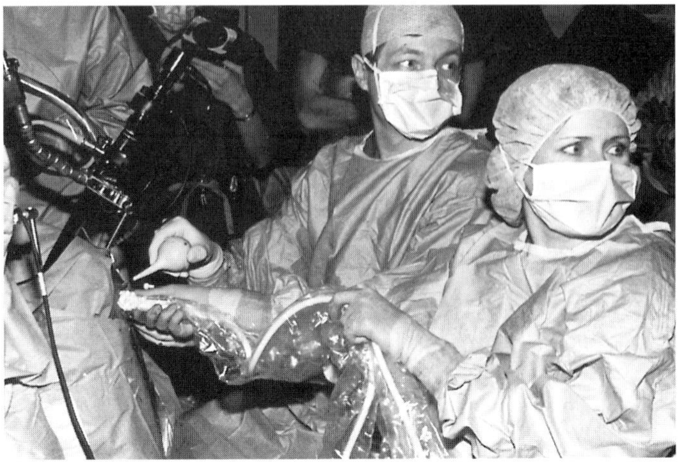

Fig. 2. Scan interface. The neurosurgeon moistens the dura or brain with sterile saline thus providing an acoustical interface with the covered transducer.

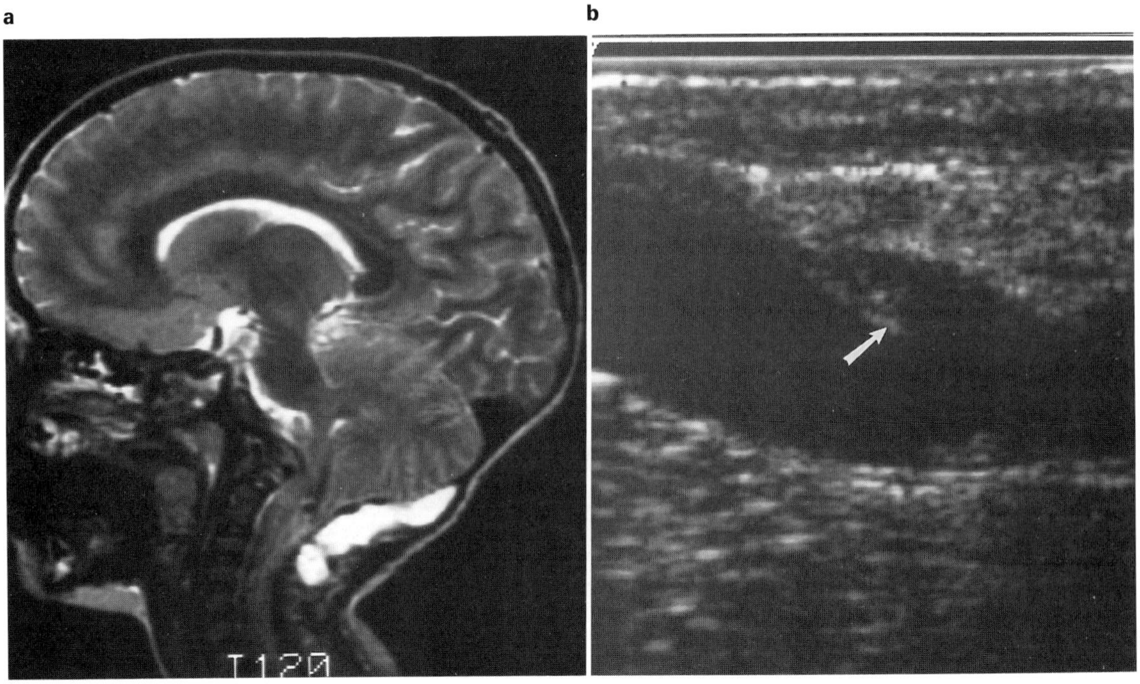

Fig. 3. Drainage guidance. **a** T2-weighted MR demonstrates a collection of high signal intensity fluid at the craniocervical junction in this patient with a surgically decompressed Chiari malformation. **b** Sagittal ultrasound image through the overlying skin demonstrates the tip of a 22 g angiocath (arrow) used to drain the extradural fluid. Note the cerebellar vermis and spinal cord deep to the collection.

lization of the radiologist's scanning arm during prolonged procedures. The neurosurgeon moistens the dura or brain parenchyma with sterile saline thus providing an acoustical interface with the covered transducer (fig. 2). When scanning the spine (patient prone) the laminectomy defect can be filled with saline and the transducer face rests on the surface.

Scanning can be performed in multiple planes through the craniotomy defect or open fontanelle. In some cases a separate burr hole may be necessary to allow optimal visualization of the tip of inserted instruments in two orthogonal planes. Operating lights must be turned down during scanning so that the video screen can be well visualized. The radiologist scans while a sonography technologist operates the controls. The neurosurgeon controls or manipulates the surgical field as necessary. The radiologist first orients him/herself to the brain anatomy, optimizes the machine settings, and then orients the neurosurgeon to the image being shown. Concise oral communication between the radiologist and neurosurgeon is important throughout the procedure. The scan time should be limited to a minimum. One must remember to take hard copy images or videotape the procedure for a permanent record.

Uses of Intraoperative Ultrasound

Guidance for Aspiration of Cysts and Other Fluid Collections

Intracranial fluid collections such as arachnoid cysts, porencephalic cysts, and postoperative fluid collections can be drained under ultrasound guidance (fig. 3). The needle or drainage catheter is readily visualized as it approaches and enters the fluid collection. Confirmation of successful drainage of the fluid collection can be made at the time of surgery decreasing the need for postoperative imaging.

Shunt Placement

Shunts are placed in pediatric patients to drain enlarged ventricles in hydrocephalus and to drain cystic masses such as arachnoid cysts or a syrinx of the spinal cord. The anterior fontanelle in the infant provides an acoustic window for visualization of the dilated ventricle and shunt catheter during placement (fig. 4). The fontanelle is outside of the sterile field and the transducer does not need to be covered in this situation. In older patients a craniotomy defect or burr hole is required. The catheter can be easily visualized and its position in the fluid collection demonstrated (fig. 4b).

Guidance of Ventriculoscopy Procedures

An increasing number of neurosurgical procedures are being performed through a ventriculoscope including biopsies, laser ablation of neoplasm and other masses, and laser fenestration of cysts. Intraoperative sonography can be used to guide the placement of the introducer and ventriculoscope and for precise guidance of the laser or forceps to the site of pathology (fig. 5, 6).

Mass Evaluation and Confirmation of Resection

Intraoperative ultrasound can be used for additional information about the character of the mass, i.e., whether

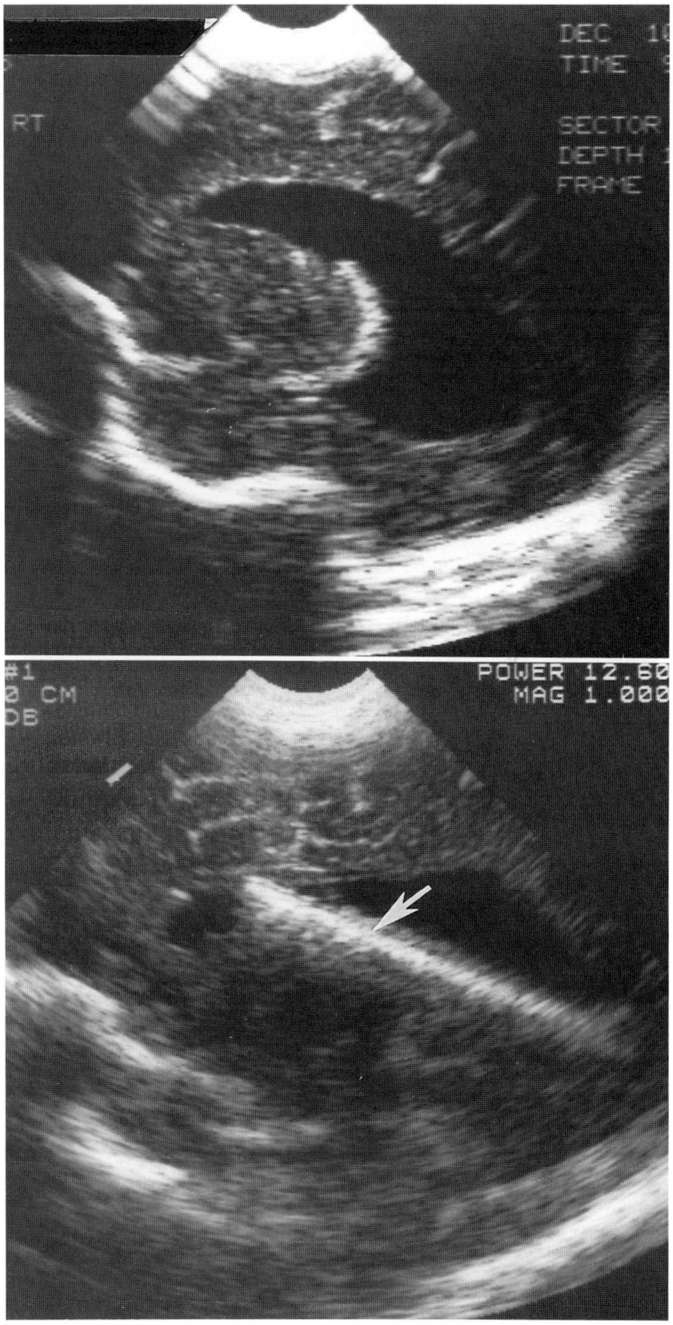

a

b

Fig. 4. Shunt placement. **a** Sagittal scan through the anterior fontanelle in an infant with Chiari II malformation demonstrates moderately dilated lateral ventricle. **b** The shunt catheter (arrow) is seen as an echogenic linear structure within the fluid-filled ventricle. Its tip in the frontal horn is confirmed.

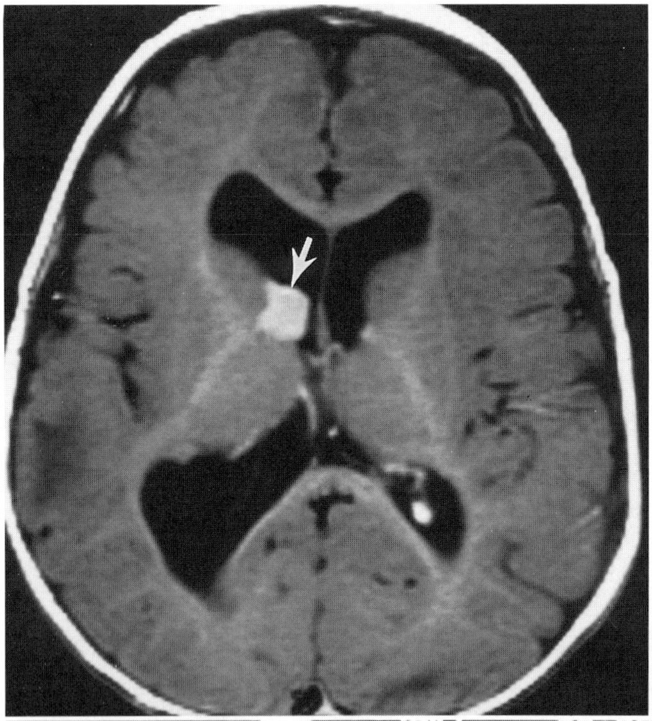

5a

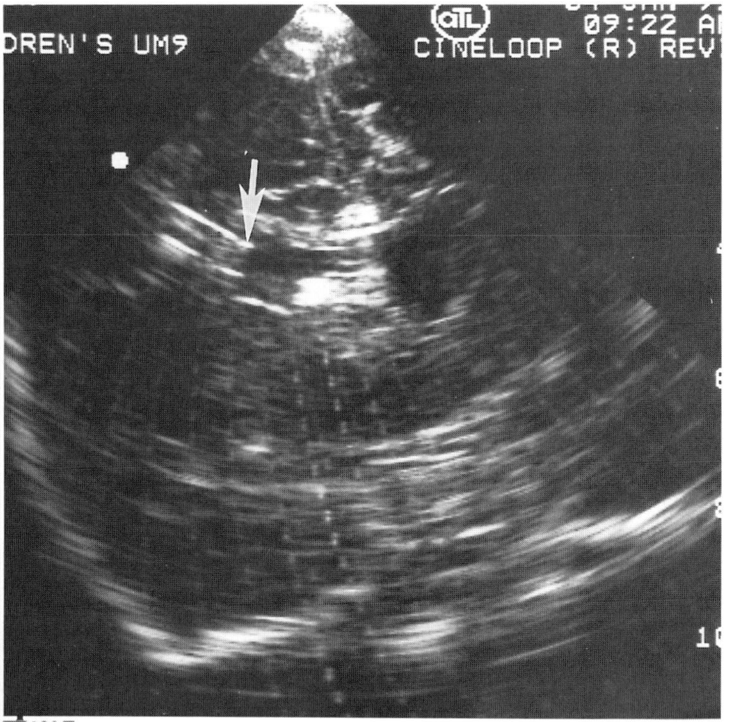

5b

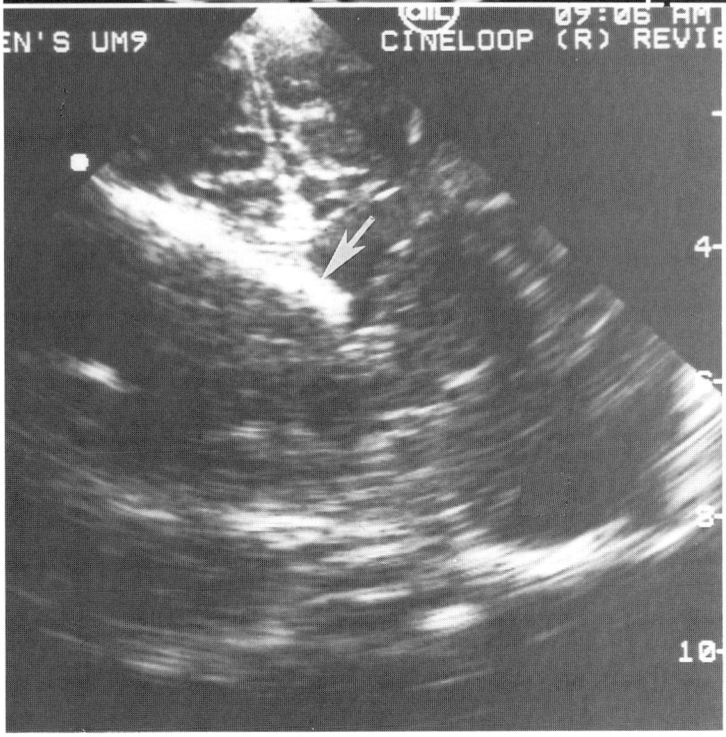

5c

Fig. 5. Biopsy guidance. **a** T1-weighted axial MR (postcontrast) demonstrates an enhancing subependymal mass (arrow) in this infant with known tuberous sclerosis. **b** Coronal sonogram. Ventriculoscope (arrow) entering the right lateral ventricle. **c** Alligator microforceps (arrow) inserted through the ventriculoscope are visualized in the coronal plane as biopsies are obtained with the transducer in the anterior fontanelle.

Fig. 6. Ventriculoscopy guidance. **a** Coronal T1-weighted MR with gadolinium enhancement shows an enhancing suprasellar pilocytic astrocytoma and moderate ventriculomegaly. **b** Coronal sonogram through a left-sided burr hole demonstrates the ventriculoscope (arrow) entering the right lateral ventricle and positioned for biopsy of the echogenic tumor. **c** Intraoperative scan demonstrates laser (arrow) fenestrating the septum pellucidum through the ventriculoscope. **d** Saline containing air bubbles has been injected into the right lateral ventricle (arrow) and is now present in the left lateral ventricle (arrowhead) indicating the ventricles are in communication. A ventriculoperitoneal shunt was then inserted into the right lateral ventricle.

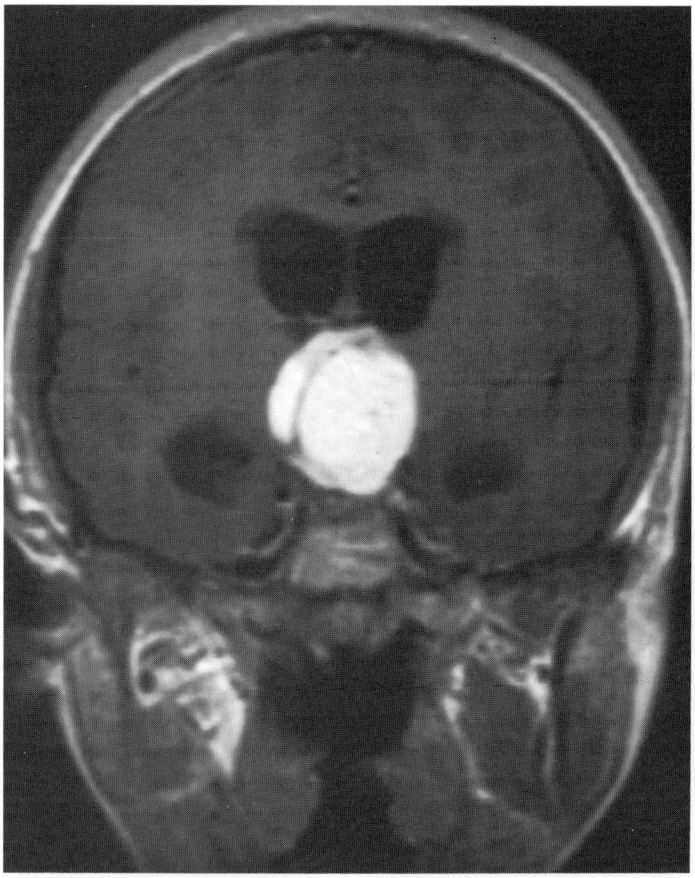

6a

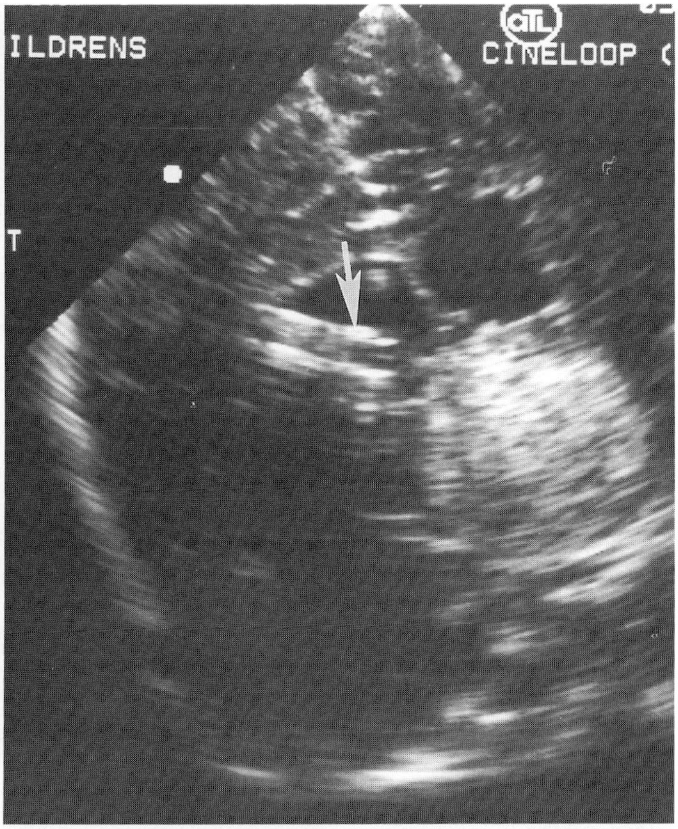

6b

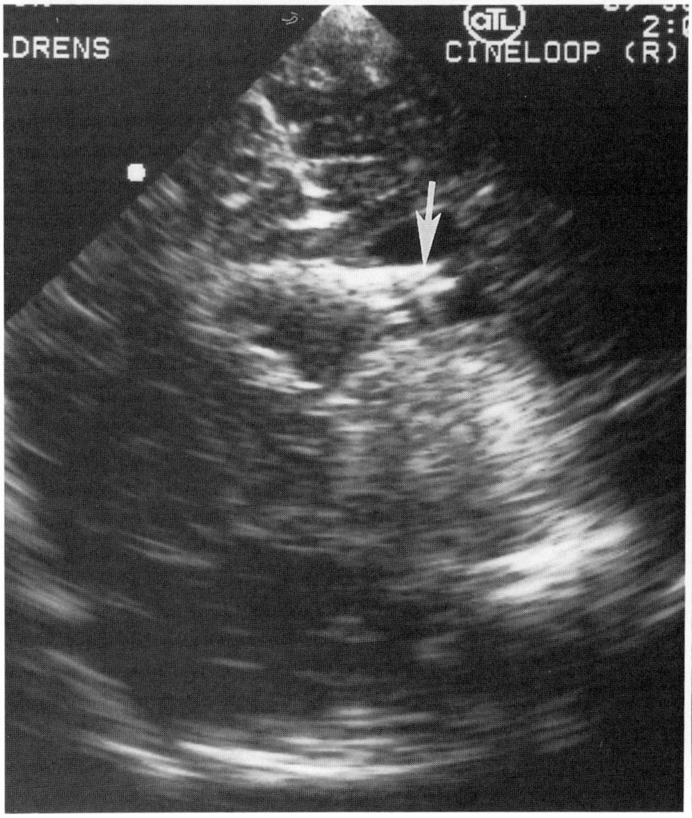

6c

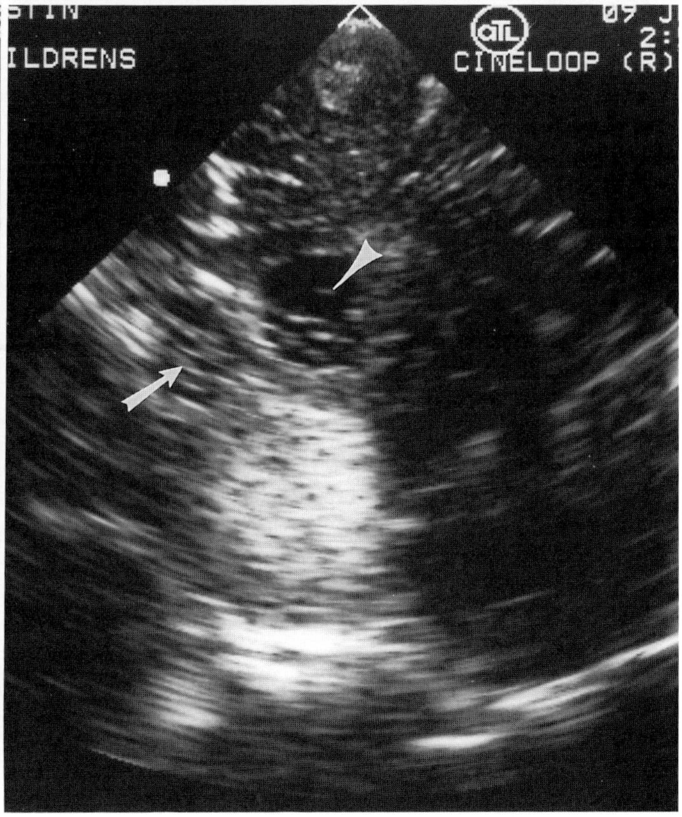

6d

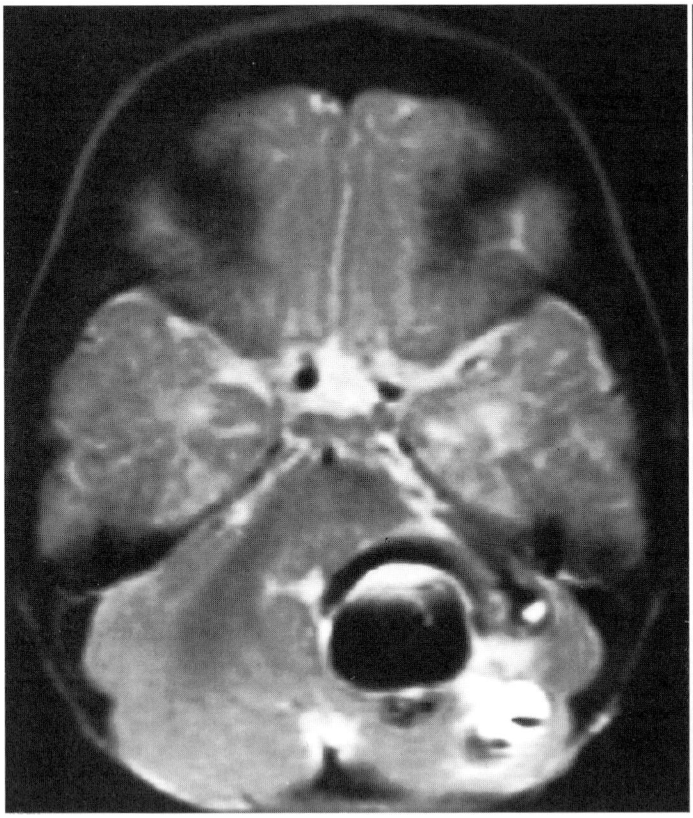

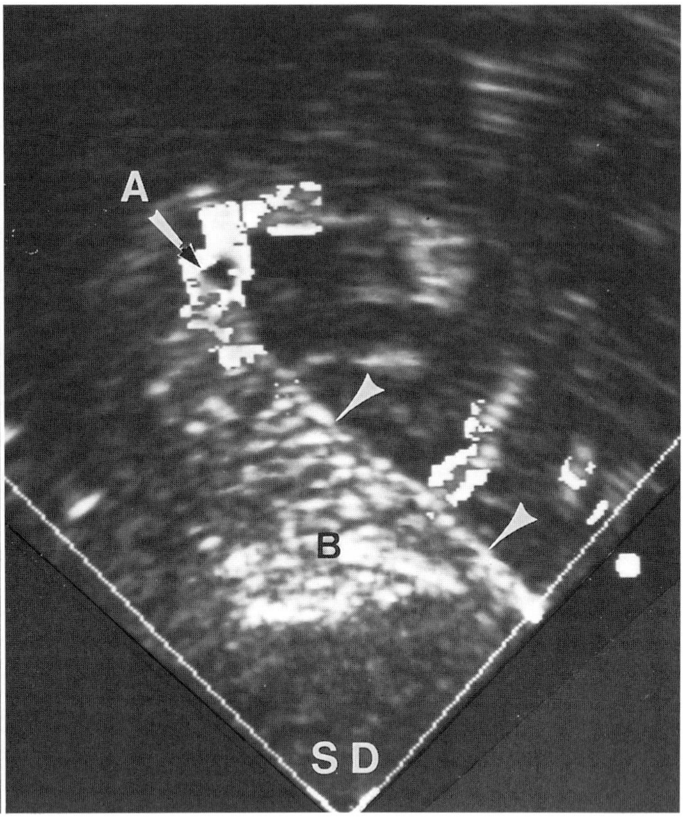

Fig. 7. Confirmation of resection. **a** Axial T2-weighted (2500/30) MR image demonstrates a mass with mixed signal intensity in the posterior fossa occupying the left cerebellar hemisphere. The center of the largest cyst has low signal intensity. The findings are consistent with a vascular malformation, but a cystic neoplasm could not be excluded. **b** Intraoperative color Doppler image has been inverted. A surgical defect (SD) in the occiput allowed scanning in the posterior fossa (the image has been inverted for correlation with MR). Abutting the tentorium (arrowheads) there is echogenic material (B) representing blood and absorbable gelatin sterile sponge in the posterior fossa. Color Doppler image permits accurate identification of the residual venous angioma (A) deep in the posterior fossa superimposed with the color map (photographed in black and white) [with permission from 9].

it is cystic or solid, and its vascularity. Sonography can also be used at the end of the procedure prior to closing to confirm complete resection of the mass (fig. 7).

Evaluation of Vascular Malformations

Intraoperative ultrasound evaluation of brain and spinal cord vascular malformations is useful for precise localization of the malformation and identification of the extent and location of the feeding arteries and draining veins. The results of preoperative embolization of the malformation can be determined and the neurosurgeon can be guided in the resection of the malformation (fig. 8). Color Doppler can also be used to confirm the completeness of the resection. It can aid in differentiation of residual malformation from hematoma and gel foam which can be difficult with B-mode scanning since all three are echogenic (fig. 8). The need for intraoperative angiography and repeat surgery for incomplete resection may be decreased.

Aneurysm Identification

Cerebral aneurysms can be identified with the use of color Doppler imaging. Intraoperative sonography has been particularly useful in the cases of aneurysms located deep within the brain and not readily visible (fig. 9). The most direct course to the aneurysm can be determined and the neurosurgeon guided to the site. After treatment, color Doppler may be used to determine whether or not the neck of an aneurysm has been adequately clipped by looking for the presence of residual blood flow.

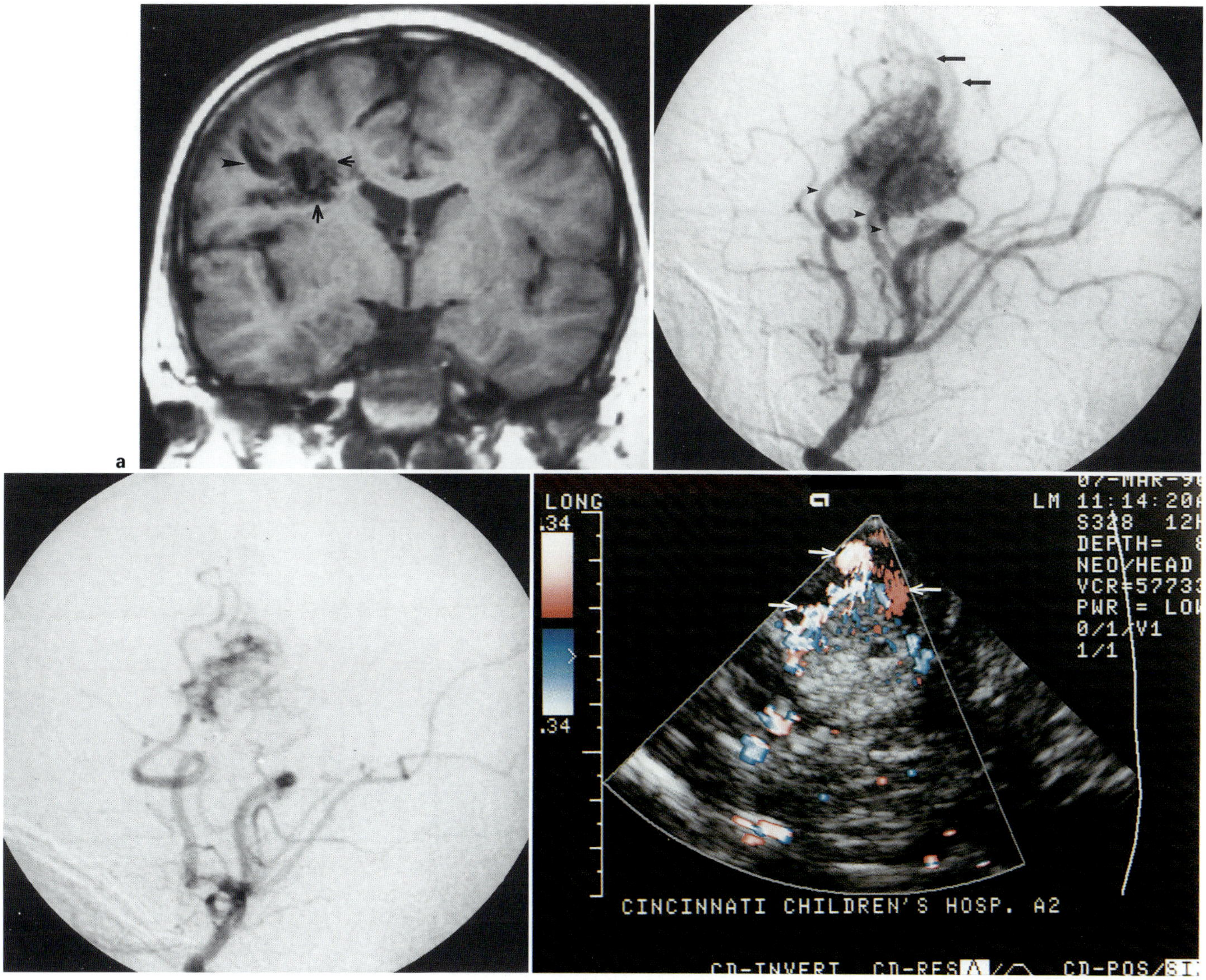

Fig. 8. Evaluation of vascular malformations. **a** Coronal T1-weighted [1,600/20 (repetition time ms/echo time ms)] MR image demonstrates flow void in a large draining vein (arrowhead) and arteries supplying the arteriovenous malformation nidus (arrows). **b** Lateral view during angiography of the right internal carotid artery after selective injection demonstrates multiple arteries (arrowheads) supplying the arteriovenous malformation. There is early filling of the draining veins (arrows). **c** Lateral view during angiography of the right internal carotid artery obtained with selective injection after embolization demonstrates decreased flow into the inferior posterior aspect of the malformation. **d** Sagittal color Doppler image obtained through the surgical defect, with the dura intact, demonstrates residual draining veins (arrows) superficial to the echogenic mass [with permission from 9].

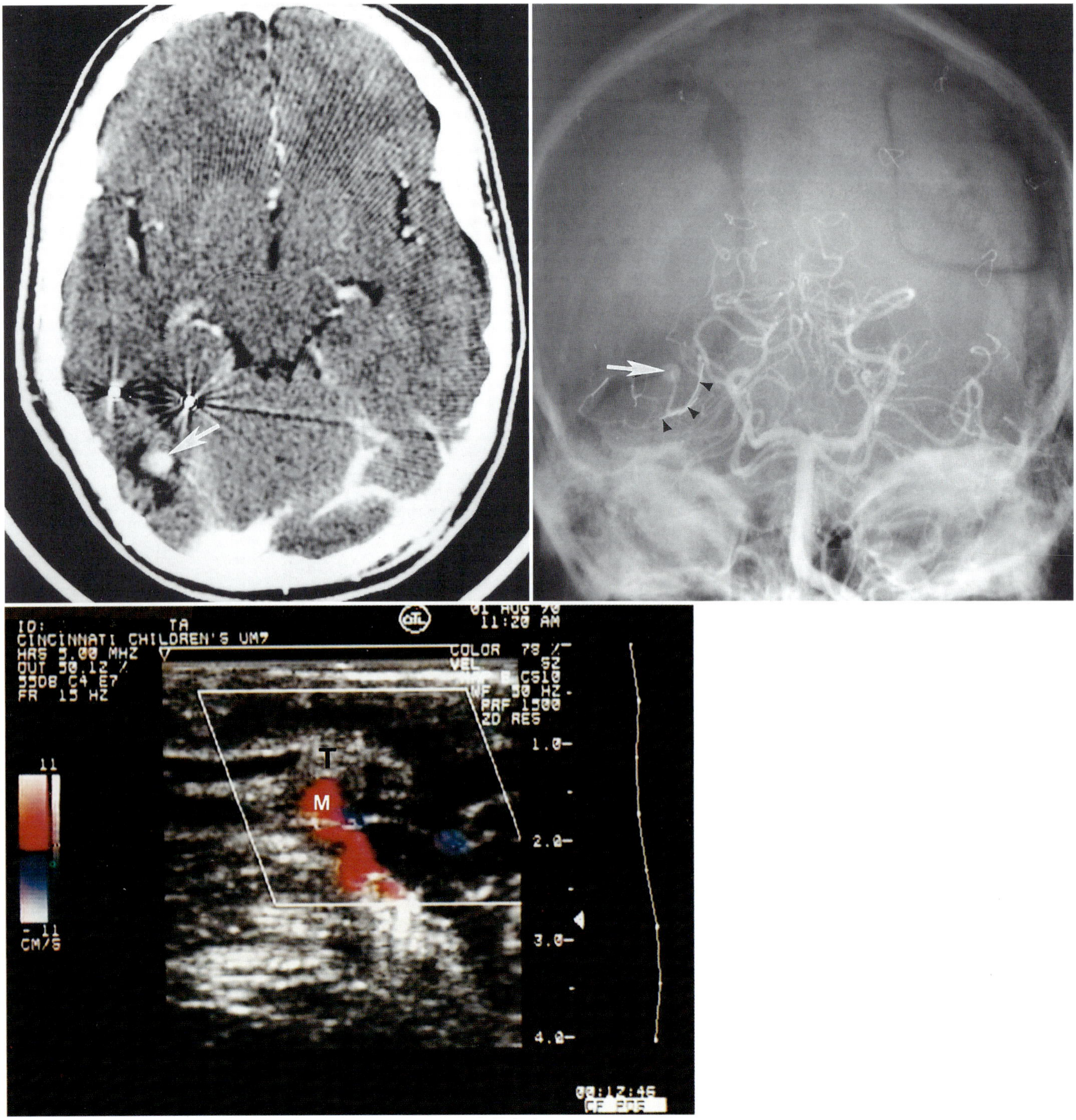

a b c

Fig. 9. Aneurysm identification. This 17-year-old with history of subacute bacterial endocarditis had three known mycotic aneurysms, with previous surgical resection of two aneurysms through two separate craniotomies. The remaining aneurysm could not be localized during the surgical procedure and thus was not resected. **a** Axial CT demonstrates location of remaining aneurysm (arrow) and artifacts from surgical clips. **b** Anterior posterior view during angiography obtained with injection into the left vertebral artery demonstrates the remaining aneurysm in the right occipital lobe (arrow) close to the surgical clips from previous aneurysm resections (arrowheads). The right calvarial flap was subsequently lifted for reoperation. **c** Axial color Doppler image obtained before the dura was opened demonstrates flow to the bulbous mycotic aneurysm (M), which lies 1.3 cm deep to the dura. A crescentic hyperechoic area (T) superficial to the flow represents the thrombosed portion of the aneurysm [with permission from 9].

Pitfalls and Limitations

Intraoperative ultrasound is presently limited to some degree by the relatively large size of the transducers presently available and the sometimes small surgical opening in the bony calvarium. Consultation between the ultrasound staff, neuroradiologists, and neurosurgeons to discuss and plan the case prior to the operative procedure minimizes this limitation. By familiarizing the neurosurgeons with the transducer sizes available, an adequate surgical window is usually possible. Manufacturers are presently developing small scan heads and the applications of intraoperative ultrasound may be expanded.

Air may get in the operative field either inadvertently or if injected by the neurosurgeon. It can obscure visualization of important anatomy and should be avoided if possible.

Doppler may not recognize all vascular masses as such because of the inability to identify small vessels (less than 0.6 mm in diameter with present equipment) or vessels with low velocity flow. Care must be taken to avoid scanning in a plane perpendicular to the vessel to be visualized since this also limits flow detection with both duplex and color Doppler.

Conclusion

Intraoperative ultrasonography has proved useful in a variety of neurosurgical and interventional procedures including shunt catheter insertion, drainage procedures, biopsy guidance and mass evaluation and confirmation of resection. Color Doppler has proved useful for precise localization of vascular lesions, selection of the shortest least vascular approach, identification of residual vascular malformation, identification of aneurysms and the confirmation of their treatment, and the evaluation of vascular tumors. Intraoperative ultrasound provides immediate ongoing information about the anatomy and flow dynamics. Pitfalls are minimal. Operating time is not significantly increased and appropriate alteration in the surgical approach is hastened. Consultation between the ultrasound staff, neuroradiologist, and neurosurgeons prior to the operative procedure maximizes the usefulness of ultrasound, thus aiding in the success of the surgery.

References

1 Chandler WF, Knake JE, McGillicuddy JE, Lillehei KO, Silver TM: Intraoperative use of real-time ultrasonography in neurosurgery. J Neurosurg 1982;57:157–163.

2 Knake JE, Chandler WF, McGillicuddy JE, Silver TM, Gabrielson TO: Intraoperative sonography for brain tumor localization and ventricular shunt placement. AJR 1982;139:733–738.

3 Rubin JM, Dohrmann GJ: Efficacy of intraoperative US for evaluating intracranial masses. Radiology 1985;157:509–511.

4 Rubin JM, DePietro MA, Chandler WF, Venes JL: Spinal ultrasonography: Intraoperative and pediatric applications. Radiol Clin North Am 1988;26:1–27.

5 Rubin JM, Hatfield MK, Chandler WF, Black KL, DiPietro MA: Intracerebral arteriovenous malformations: Intraoperative color Doppler flow imaging. Radiology 1989;170:219–222.

6 Black KL, Rubin JM, Chandler WF, McGillicuddy JE: Intraoperative color-flow Doppler imaging of AVM's and aneurysms. J Neurosurg 1988;68:635–639.

7 Nornes H, Grip A, Wikeby P: Intraoperative evaluation of cerebral hemodynamics using directional Doppler technique. J Neurosurg 1979;50:145–151.

8 Rubin JM, Knake JE: Intraoperative sonography of a spinal cord arteriovenous malformation. AJNR 1987;8:730–731.

9 Barr LL, Babcock DS, Crone KR, Berger TS, Ball WS, Prenger EC: Color Doppler US imaging during pediatric neurosurgical and neuroradiologic procedures. Radiology 1991;181:567–571.

Pediatr Neurosurg 1992;18:92–104

Richard R. Smith

Department of Radiology and Neurology, Indiana University School of Medicine, Indianapolis, Ind., USA

Neuroradiology of Intracranial Infection

Key Words
Brain
Meninges
Infection
Inflammation
Magnetic resonance imaging

Abstract
The ability to detect and differentiate intracranial infection has markedly improved, first with the introduction of computed tomography and, more recently, with magnetic resonance. Enhanced magnetic resonance imaging is the procedure of choice in the evaluation of nearly all intracranial infections. The sensitivity of MR to foci of increased water content, seen in most parenchymal infections, the lack of bone artifact, and the multiplanar capability of MR have led to this preeminence. Computed tomography remains useful primarily in those infections associated with intracranial calcification, such as TORCH syndrome. This article summarizes the most recent CT and MR findings of infection involving the meninges and brain parenchyma.

Introduction

The introduction of magnetic resonance imaging (MRI) in the last decade revolutionized neuroradiology in general. More specifically, the ability to detect intracranial infection on MR was found to be superior to that of computed tomography (CT) [1, 2]. Not only did MRI improve the detection of infectious lesions not identified on routine CT, it also better demonstrated the extent and improved the specificity of lesions that were seen on CT. This superiority is primarily because MRI is more sensitive to alterations in brain water content, a condition seen in nearly all parenchymal infections. The lack of bone artifacts led to improved sensitivity to lesions in the temporal lobes and posterior fossa, as well as the detection of meningeal inflammation. The multiplanar capability of MR led to improved evaluation of the extent of lesions, both, for therapeutic planning and in evaluating therapeutic efficacy. These advantages of MRI have led to this modality becoming the procedure of choice in the evaluation of intracranial infection.

An appropriate MRI strategy should consist of nonenhanced short TR (T1-weighted) and nonenhanced long TR (T2-weighted) images. Following the administration of gadolinium (Gd), an MRI contrast agent, a series of T1-weighted images should be performed. Contrast enhancement in MR depends upon localized shortening of T1 values as opposed to increased electron density with CT imaging. The distribution of contrast, however, is similar to that of CT, with areas of blood brain barrier breakdown, and to a lesser degree, areas of intrinsic vascularity showing contrast enhancement.

Meningitis and Complications

Meningitis

Most clinical cases of meningitis are either bacterial or viral. With the increased number of AIDS cases, the incidence of fungal meningitis is also increasing. Other miscellaneous infectious causes include tuberculosis and syphilis. Most cases of adult meningitis are the result of

Richard R. Smith, MD
Department of Radiology
University Hospital, Room 0279
926 West Michigan Street
Indianapolis, IN 46202-5253 (USA)

1016–2291/92/0182–0092
$2.75/0

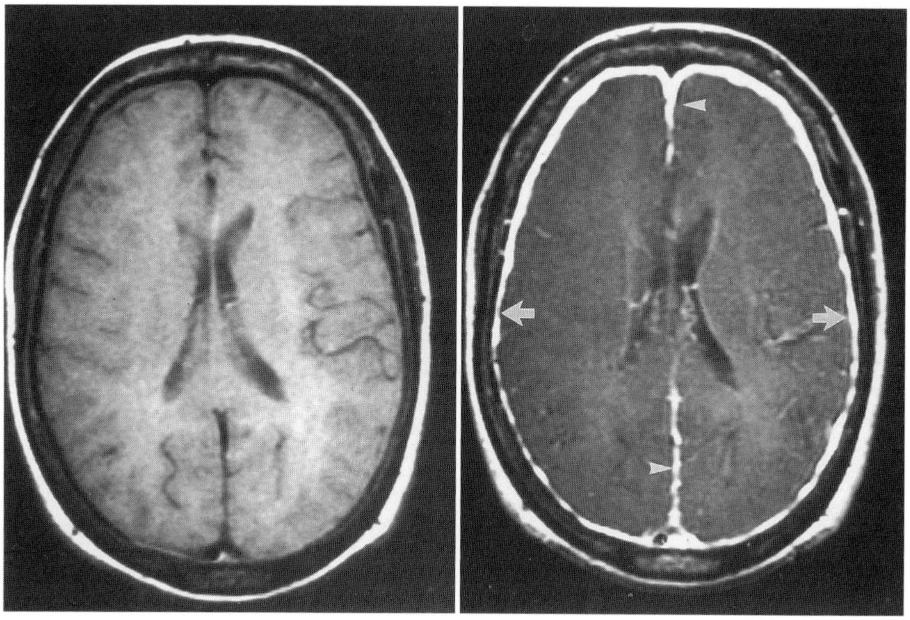

Fig. 1. Pneumococcal meningitis. Axial nonenhanced (**a**) and gadolinium-enhanced (**b**) T1-weighted images through the level of the lateral ventricles demonstrate changes secondary to diffuse meningitis. The unenhanced study is normal. The enhanced image demonstrates bilateral convexity (arrows) and falcine (arrowheads) enhancement.

hematogenous spread from an area of active infection elsewhere in the body. In children many cases are secondary to contiguous spread from either paranasal sinus or middle ear inflammatory disease.

Before the introduction of MR, CT was used in cases of meningitis primarily to exclude mass lesions precluding lumbar puncture or in the evaluation of secondary complications. Most CT studies in patients with meningitis are normal [3]. If abnormal, the CT study typically demonstrates abnormal enhancement within the basal cisterns, and to a lesser degree in the fissures and sulci. Convexity dural enhancement is difficult to appreciate because of the adjacent dense bone.

With the introduction of contrast-enhanced MRI, the ability to detect meningitis has improved. Normally, the meninges show no enhancement or subtle thin focal areas of dural enhancement on T1-weighted images following Gd administration. Meningitis is usually associated with marked dural enhancement (fig. 1). The enhancement may involve the basal cisterns, fissures and sulci, but is usually most evident along the falx cerebri, tentorium and convexity dura. The enhancement is usually contiguous and linear. Noncontrast T1- and T2-weighted images are usually normal.

There have been few reports of the actual incidence of abnormal meningeal enhancement in meningitis. In a report by Chang et al. [2], only 10 of 18 patients, with a variety of etiologies of meningitis showed abnormal enhancement. In fact, in that study, no patient with viral meningitis demonstrated abnormal MR enhancement. This trend is similar to another study by Mathews et al. [4] which demonstrated an increased sensitivity to bacterial meningitis as opposed to viral meningitis.

Care should be taken in the evaluation of abnormal meningeal enhancement, however. This finding is not specific for infectious meningitis. In fact, abnormal meningeal enhancement can be seen in a variety of other disease states, including carcinomatous meningitis, inflammatory sarcoidosis, after subarachnoid hemorrhage and after ventriculoperitoneal shunt placement. MRI, therefore, should not be used as the primary method of diagnosis of meningitis. MRI may be useful to rule out mass lesions and to provide further evidence of meningeal inflammation in atypical clinical cases or in cases where CSF results are not clear-cut.

Meningitis Complications

There are a variety of complications associated with meningitis including hydrocephalus, extra-axial fluid collections, infarction, venous thrombosis and ventriculitis.

Communicating hydrocephalus is the most common complication associated with meningitis. The etiology is related to inflammatory debris obstructing the flow and resorption of CSF, particularly at the arachnoid villi. If obstruction occurs within the cerebral aqueduct or along the outflow of the fourth ventricle, an obstructive component of hydrocephalus can be seen. Communicating hydrocephalus generally manifests itself with an increase in

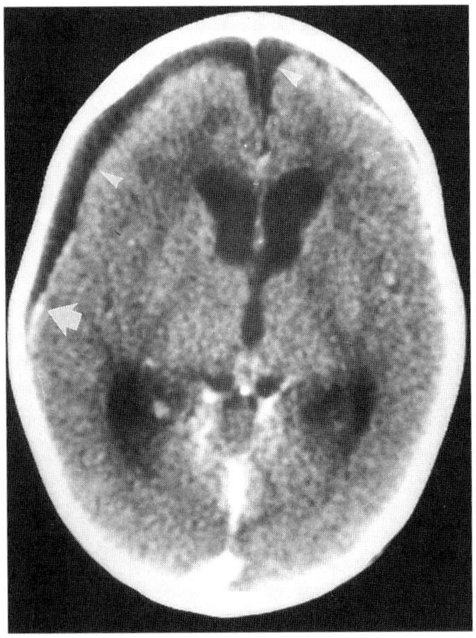

Fig. 2. Communicating hydrocephalus and subdural effusion. Axial contrast-enhanced CT scan demonstrates ventricular enlargement. Subdural effusions are seen bilaterally (arrowheads). A small amount of abnormal meningeal enhancement is seen (arrow) along the right cerebral convexity, consistent with meningitis.

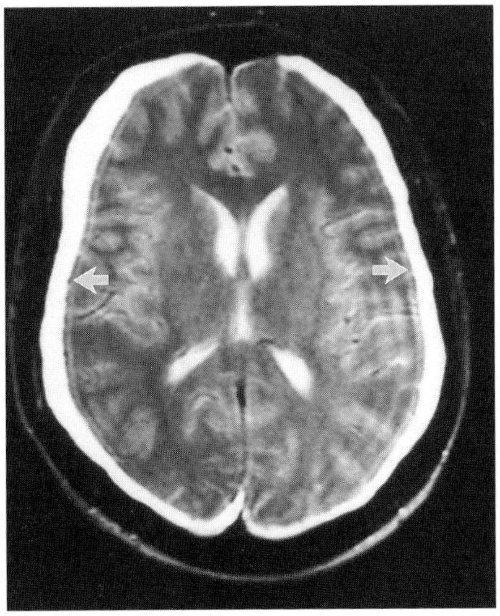

Fig. 3. H. flu subdural effusion. Bilateral high signal effusions (arrows) are seen on this T2-weighted image. No underlying parenchymal abnormality is seen.

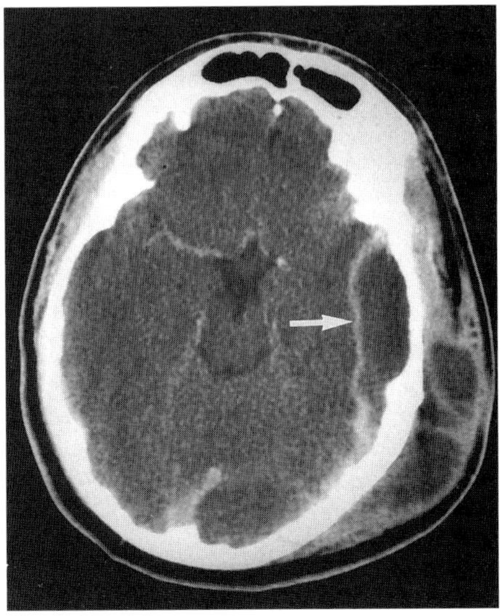

Fig. 4. Epidural abscess. Axial contrast-enhanced CT scan demonstrates a large left temporal epidural abscess. The enhancing dural margin is seen along the medial aspect of the abscess (arrow). A large subgaleal collection of purulent material is also seen. This collection was secondary to untreated bacterial mastoiditis.

ventricular (fig. 2) and sulcal prominence, abnormal for age. Symptoms referable to hydrocephalus are frequently present and ventricular decompression may be necessary.

Extra-axial collections associated with meningitis may be infected or sterile. The most frequent collection is a sterile subdural effusion. Presumably these effusions are secondary to irritation of the dura due to the infected subarachnoid fluid [5]. These collections are typically isointense to CSF on both CT (fig. 3) and on all imaging sequences in MR. There is a notable lack of underlying parenchymal abnormality. These subdural collections can become infected if there is rupture of the arachnoid or a ruptured infected vein in the subdural space. Such a collection, a subdural empyema, may have a higher signal intensity than CSF both on CT and on all imaging MRI pulse sequences secondary to increased protein content within the infected collection. There is often a more severe underlying inflammation of the brain parenchyma, typically better seen on MR than on CT. Epidural abscess associated with meningitis is most frequently seen in those cases that result from direct extension. They are most often found adjacent to the sphenoethmoid sinus or in the vicinity of the mastoid and middle ear cavity. Epidural abscesses may be associated with penetrating trauma. As in cases of subdural empyema, the signal intensity within the collection is usually higher than that of CSF on both CT and MR (fig. 4). The dura is thickened and shows marked enhancement following contrast administration (fig. 4). The underlying brain parenchyma is usually normal, the dura acting as a strong barrier against further intracranial spread. MR is more sensitive in the detection of thin collections along the convexity or along the base of the brain [6].

Infarction associated with meningitis occurs either because of an inflammatory-induced arterial spasm or because of direct invasion of arteries and arterioles. Most infarcts are found to occur in the basal ganglia, secondary to spasm or occlusion of penetrating lenticulostriate arteries. Large branch occlusions can result in cortical infarction. At times it may be difficult to differentiate a meningitic-associated infarct from adjacent encephalitis. Both entities will show low density with patchy enhancement on CT. On MRI, such lesions will demonstrate sulcal effacement with mass effect. Although T1-weighted images may demonstrate subtle hypointensity, T2-

a b

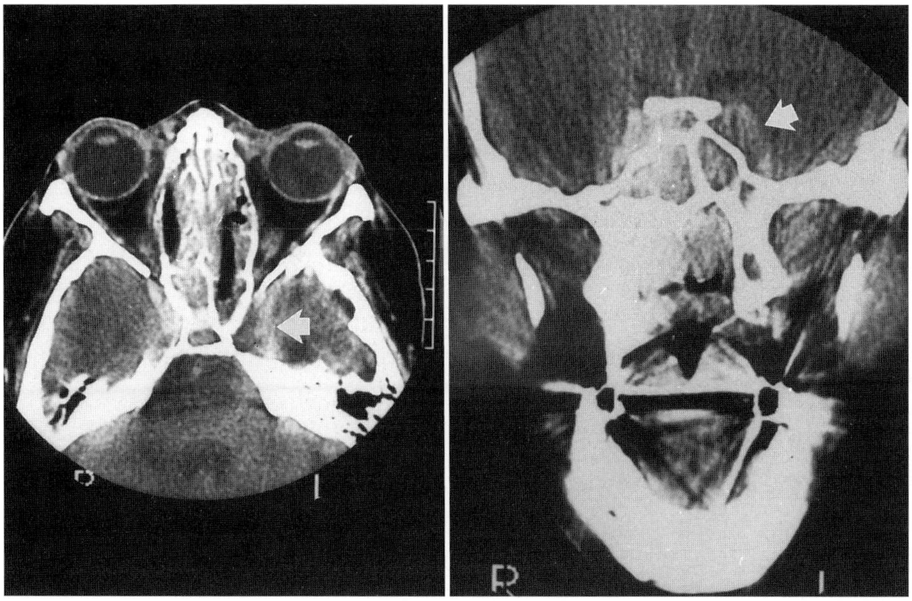

Fig. 5a, b. Fungal cavernous sinus thrombosis. Axial and coronal postcontrast CT scans demonstrate enlargement and abnormal decreased intensity within the left cavernous sinus (arrows). The coronal view demonstrates a convex outer margin of the left cavernous sinus. There is complete opacification of the sphenoid sinus with postoperative changes in the ethmoid sinuses. There was associated meningitis, clinically, as well.

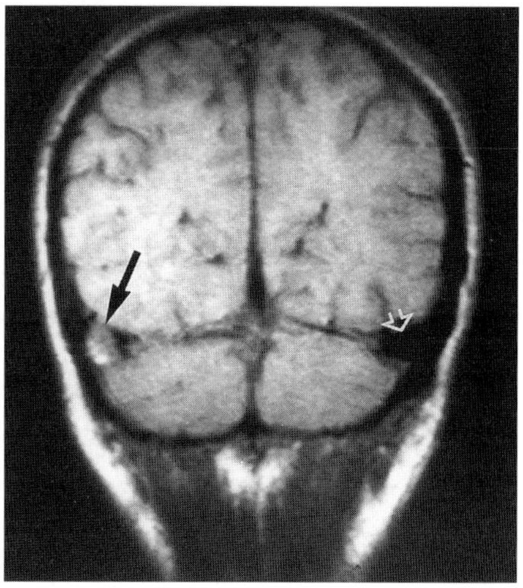

Fig. 6. Dural sinus thrombosis. Coronal T1-weighted image shows loss of flow void in the right, transverse sinus (closed arrow). The left transverse sinus is patent as shown by the preserved flow void (open arrow). Patient with otitic meningitis.

weighted images are more likely to demonstrate increased signal intensity. Gadolinium enhancement may be seen in a patchy distribution, and in infarction there may also be intra-arterial vascular enhancement [7].

Venous thrombosis can affect either cortical veins or dural sinuses. Unenhanced CT may demonstrate an increased intravascular density. With contrast administration there is a relatively greater enhancement of the margins of dural sinus as opposed to the thrombosed contents (fig. 5). This results in the so-called ‘delta sign’. With MRI, moderate to rapidly flowing blood is hypointense, resulting in a normal signal void. With venous or dural thrombosis there is a loss of flow void (fig. 6). MR has significantly improved the detection of dural sinus and cortical venous thrombosis. Gadolinium administration results in the same ‘delta sign’, with enhancement of the margins of the sinus but without enhancement of the central thrombosed lumen [8].

Ventriculitis may be seen in association with meningitis, secondary to rupture of a parenchymal abscess into the ventricles or may occur following catheter placement. On CT, there may be some low density along the ventricular margins, and with contrast there will be enhancement along the ventricular wall. On T2-weighted MR images there is abnormal increased signal intensity in the periventricular region. Following gadolinium administration on T1-weighted images, there is marked periventricular enhancement. Associated choroid plexitis may also be seen [9].

Cerebritis and Abscess

Cerebritis and abscess may have a variety of causes. In children many cases are secondary to direct extension from the middle ear or secondary to hematogenous spread in congenital heart disease. In adults, these infections are most likely related to areas of suppuration elsewhere in the body with hematogenous spread. Penetrating trauma in young adults is also a frequent cause of cerebritis and/or abscess. Most abscesses that are hematogenous are identified in the gray white junction, predominately within the middle cerebral artery distribution. Hematogenous lesions are also more likely to be multiple.

The CT progression of cerebritis and abscess was first described, in detail, by Enzmann et al. [10]. In the cerebri-

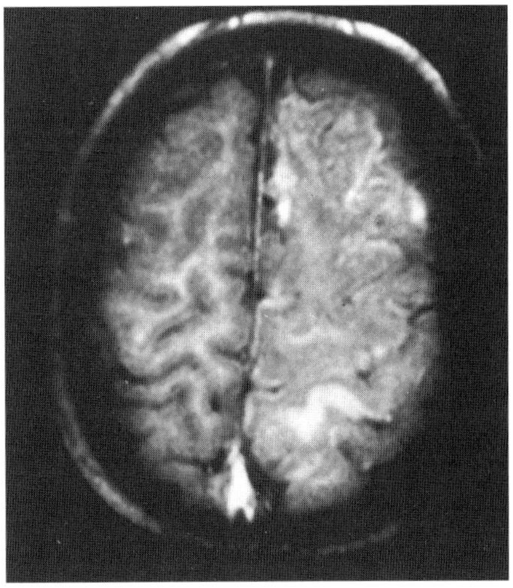

Fig. 7. Cerebritis. Axial gadolinium-enhanced T1-weighted image demonstrates mass effect with swelling of the gyri in the left cerebrum. There is abnormal enhancement within the gyri and along the pia arachnoid. The right side is normal.

tis phase, CT demonstrates parenchymal low density. There is frequently mass effect as evidenced by ventricular compression, or more commonly, sulcal effacement. With contrast administration there is patchy enhancement in the affected area. As the brain attempts to encapsulate the infection, a capsule of collagen and granulation tissue is formed. Ultimately the central portion will undergo necrosis. As the abscess develops, the CT appearance changes to a ring-enhancing lesion. Early in the abscess phase the central portion of the abscess may fill in with contrast on delayed imaging. In the late stage of abscess, the central portion will be necrotic, full of purulent debris, and will not fill in with contrast. The margins of the abscess capsule are frequently uniform in thickness and smooth along the inner margin. There may be a slight increased thickness of the abscess along the gray matter surface secondary to the increased blood flow. Significant mass effect and surrounding vasogenic edema are often present.

The MR appearance of cerebritis and abscess is similar to that seen with CT. The T1-weighted images are usually more sensitive in demonstrating the sulcal effacement and mass effect associated with early cerebritis. T2-weighted images show the increased water content associated with cerebritis as an increased signal intensity. With intravenous contrast patchy enhancement along the sulci and gray matter is noted (fig. 7). As the frank abscess develops, the central portion becomes hypointense on the T1-weighted image and hyperintense on the T2-weighted image. The abscess capsule frequently has a hyperintense rim on noncontrast T1-weighted images and a hypointense rim on T2-weighted images (fig. 8). This probably relates to the paramagnetic effect of free radicals within the abscess wall [11]. Some investigators have suggested, however, that this represents a small amount of hemorrhage from friable granulation tissue [12]. Evidence of vasogenic edema is well depicted on the long TR images. With contrast administration there is enhancement of the abscess capsule (fig. 8c). As with CT scanning, the capsule is relatively thin and uniform with smooth inner margins.

Viral Infections

Herpes Encephalitis

The detection of herpes encephalitis is one area where MRI has made tremendous impact. Since prognosis is directly related to the institution of early treatment, the ability of MR to detect herpes at an earlier stage than CT has led to this modality becoming the procedure of choice [13].

The type and location of herpes encephalitis is associated with the patient's age. Congenital herpes, part of the TORCH syndrome, is a systemic disease that results in microcephaly, lesions throughout the brain and foci of calcification. As with other congenital intracranial infections, however, CT is of greater sensitivity in the detection of foci of calcification than is MRI. The utility of gradient echo imaging in the detection of calcification is superior to spin echo imaging. Herpes simplex encephalitis in the older child and adult most often affects the temporal lobes and insular cortex. This specific involvement may be related to the virus remaining in a latent state within the trigeminal ganglia, and with reactivation, the virus migrates along fibers innervating the meninges and middle cranial fossa [14]. Pathologically, the infection is a hemorrhagic necrotizing encephalitis.

CT imaging may demonstrate areas of low density in the temporal lobes. Sensitivity in this area is poor, however, secondary to bone artifacts. As the infection becomes subacute, foci of hemorrhage may be seen within the temporal lobes. Contrast administration reveals a patchy enhancement within the affected areas.

MRI is of greater sensitivity not only because of its superior ability to detect edema associated with early infection, but also because of the lack of bone artifact. On nonenhanced MRI there will be evidence of mass effect

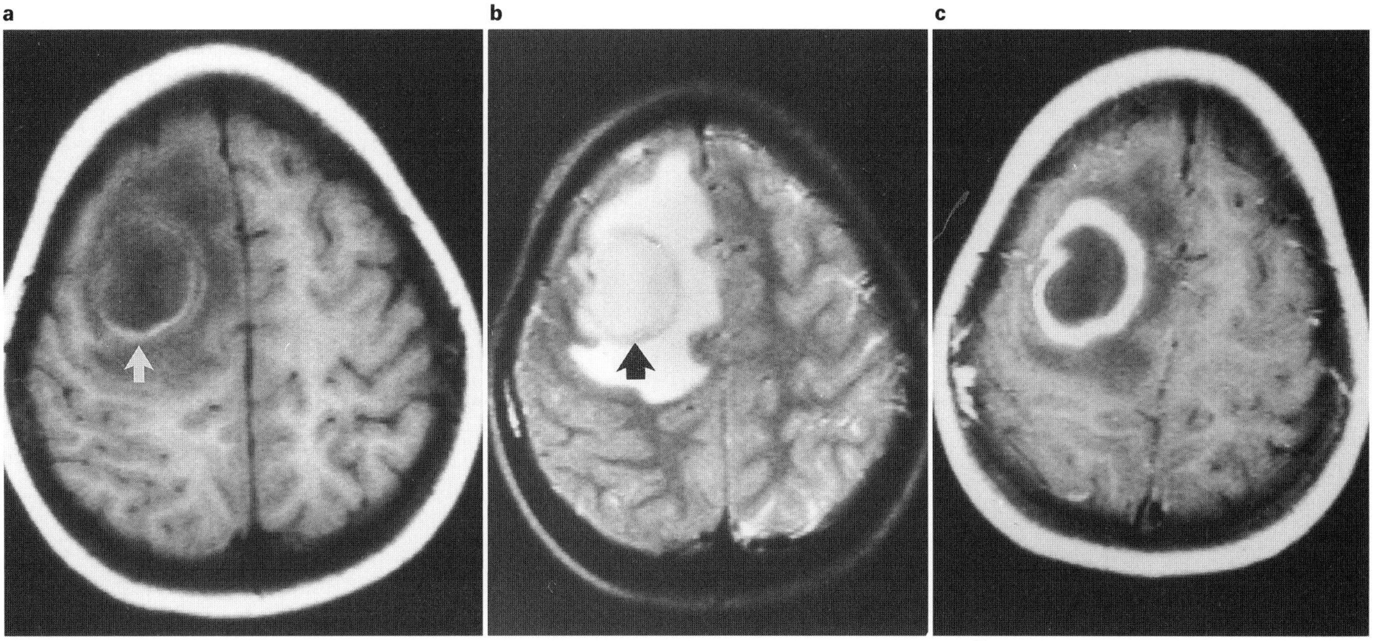

Fig. 8a–c. Abscess. Axial T1-weighted image (**a**) demonstrates decreased signal intensity within the right frontal lobe. A ring of abnormal increased signal intensity is noted (arrow). The T2-weighted image demonstrates marked edema as well as a thin rim of decreased signal intensity (arrow) corresponding with the abscess capsule. With gadolinium administration (**c**) the T1-weighted image demonstrates a mature abscess capsule. The margins are thin and uniform. The inner lining is relatively smooth.

within the temporal lobes and insular cortex. On T2-weighted images the area will have hyperintense signals (fig. 9). Foci of hemorrhage will demonstrate signal intensities associated with the stage of hemorrhage present within the lesion [15]. Areas of deoxyhemoglobin will appear as patchy areas of decreased signal intensity on T2-weighted images. Areas of methemoglobin will be hyperintense on T1-weighted images. With intravenous contrast, patchy enhancement will be seen within the temporal lobes. Coronal views are helpful in the evaluation of insular and temporal lobe involvement.

Acute Disseminated Encephalomyelitis

Acute disseminated encephalomyelitis is a postvaccinial or postinfectious demyelinating disease seen most frequently in children. The demyelination is presumed to be secondary to an autoimmune phenomenon. These patients become neurologically symptomatic approximately 1–2 weeks following vaccination or a viral-like illness such as occurs with chicken pox. Seizures and ataxia are frequent clinical presentations. Most cases will have spontaneous resolution, in some after a prolonged course. Fatalities are reported. Response to corticosteroid therapy is usually prompt and significant.

As with the detection of multiple sclerosis, demyelinating lesions within the white matter are difficult to see on CT. If present, they may be seen as vague areas of decreased attenuation in the periventricular and deep white matter. MRI is the imaging procedure of choice [16]. Multiple areas of abnormal increased signal intensity are found in the periventricular and deep white matter on T2-weighted images (fig. 10). There is usually little mass effect. Abnormal signal may also be seen in the gray matter, especially the thalami. If gadolinium is administered in the acute phase some lesions show inhomogeneous enhancement [17]. Follow-up studies often demonstrate resolution of the lesions.

Cytomegalovirus

Congenital cytomegalovirus infection is part of the TORCH syndrome. Approximately 10% of the patients with this congenital infection will have neurologic abnormalities. These consist of seizures, mental retardation and hearing and visual disturbances. There is an association with abnormal brain development including polymicrogyria and pachygyria.

CT examination is probably the procedure of choice in the detection of congenital CMV. This is primarily be-

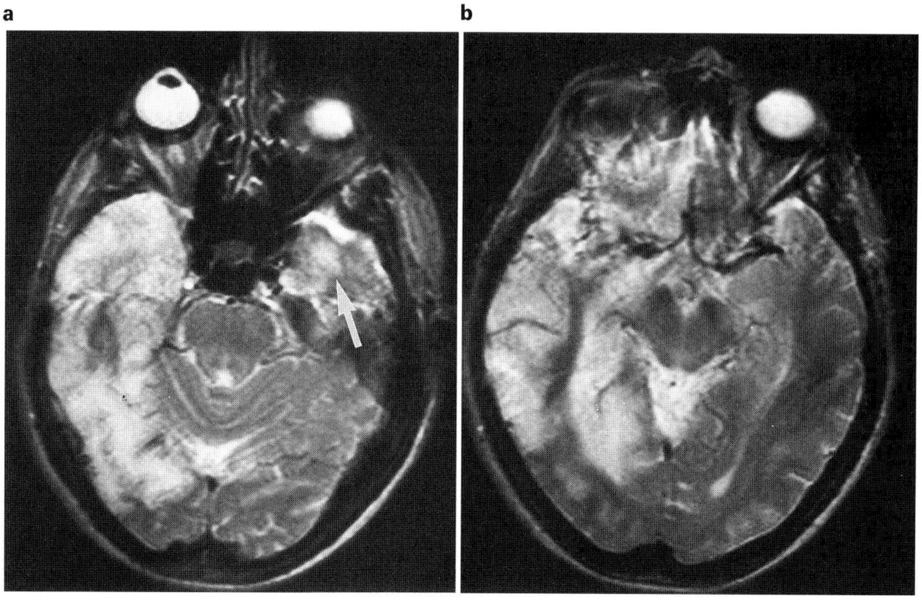

Fig. 9a, b. Herpes encephalitis. Axial T2-weighted images demonstrate prominent signal abnormality in the right temporal lobe. A smaller focus is also seen in the left temporal lobe (arrow).

10

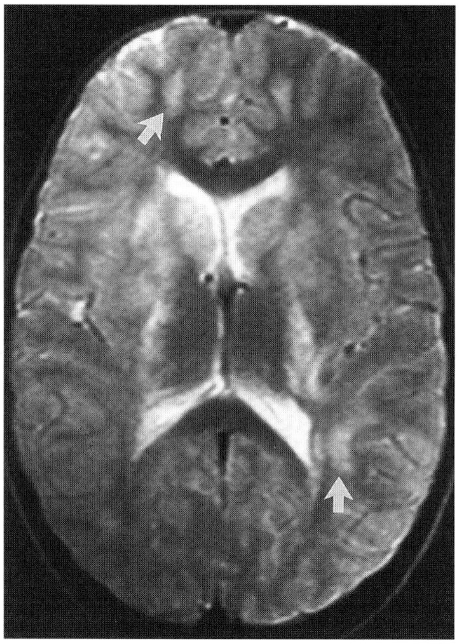

11

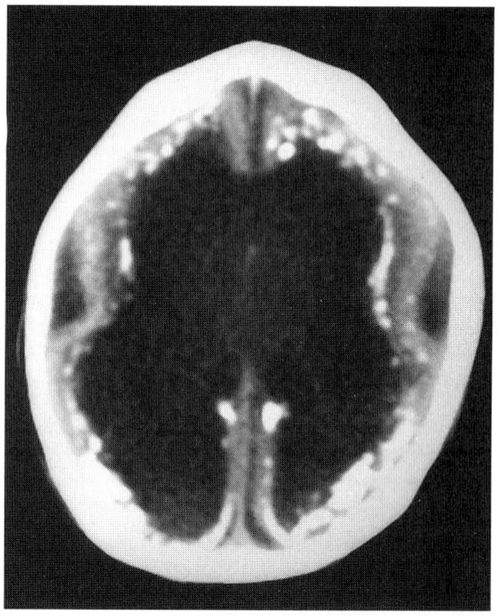

Fig. 10. Acute disseminated encephalomyelitis. Axial T2-weighted image demonstrates abnormal increased signal intensity within the right caudate head as well as extending along the lateral aspect of both thalami. Some periatrial and subcortical lesions are noted (arrows).

Fig. 11. Congenital cytomegalovirus infection. Axial nonenhanced CT scan demonstrates marked periventricular calcification. There is severe parenchymal loss. There is also associated pachygyria.

cause the hallmark of this infection, subependymal calcification, is best identified on CT (fig. 11). On MRI, such subependymal calcifications may, rarely, be demonstrated as focal areas of signal loss on T2-weighted images. Gradient echo images may be helpful in the detection of such lesions. Although CT may be the best modality for the detection of these calcifications, MRI is a complementary study as it is better at demonstrating the developmental brain abnormalities.

Fungal Infections

A wide range of fungi can cause intracranial infection. Most lesions are seen in the immunocompromised host or are associated with massive inoculation. The form that the fungus takes within the host produces different lesions [18]. Fungi that exist in hyphal forms within the host frequently cause obstruction of arteries and produce septic infarcts. Aspergillus is an example of this type of fungus.

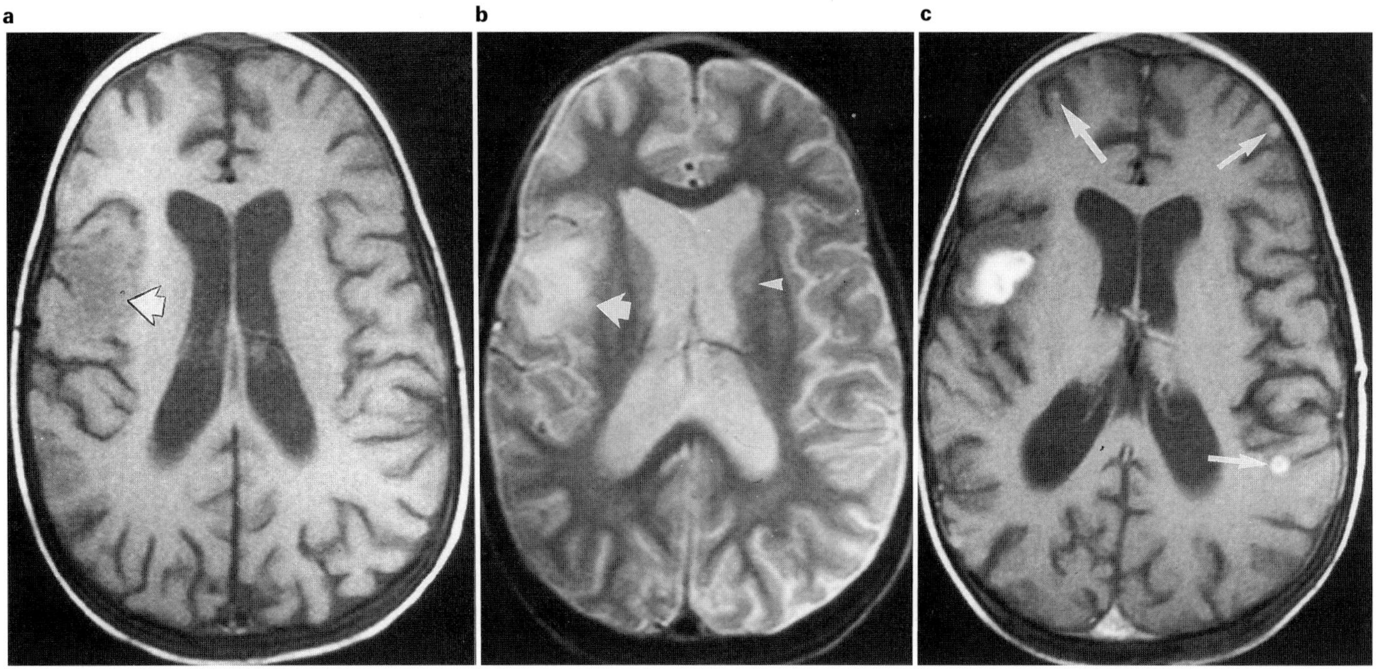

Fig. 12. Aspergillosis. Axial unenhanced T1 (**a**) and T2 (**b**) weighted images demonstrate abnormal signal intensity within the right frontoparietal lobe (arrows). The T2-weighted image also demonstrates an abnormal focus of increased signal intensity within the left caudate (arrowhead). Following gadolinium administration the T1-weighted image (**c**) demonstrates abnormal enhancement in the right frontoparietal region. Three other foci of abnormal enhancement are identified (arrows). The lesion in the left caudate was seen on the next higher slice as a small ring-enhancing nodule (not shown).

Fungi that exist as yeasts, such as cryptococcus, are able to get into small vessels resulting in meningeal or subarachnoid space infections. Fungi that exist as pseudohyphae occlude arterioles resulting in small parenchymal abscesses; candidiasis is an example of this form of infection.

Aspergillus infection of the brain is usually secondary to hematogenous spread from a pulmonary infection. The fungus invades large arteries resulting in ischemic septic infarction (fig. 12). Abscesses may be identified, with most aspergillus infections showing extensive edema and ring enhancing lesions. The appearance, however, is not specific for aspergillosis.

Cryptococcosis is now seen most commonly in patients with AIDS. Meningitis is the most frequent manifestation. Up to 70% of autopsy examinations demonstrate cryptococcal meningitis. Contrast-enhanced MR typically shows abnormal meningeal enhancement particularly in the sylvian fissures and basal cisterns (fig. 13). Small foci of cryptococcal infection have been identified within the basal ganglia in patients with AIDS. These lesions are hyperintense on T2-weighted images. The

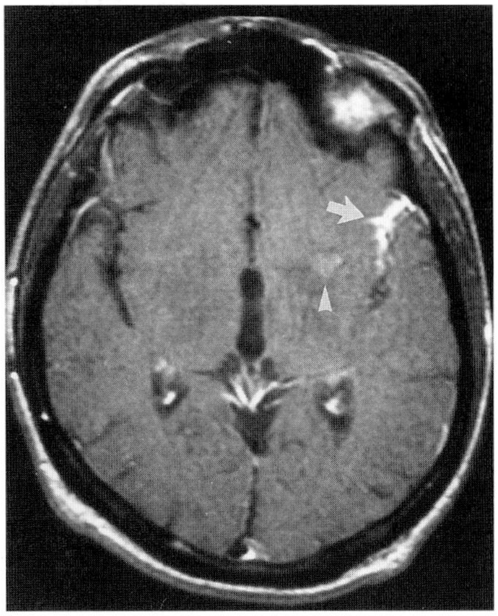

Fig. 13. AIDS-related cryptococcosis. The axial enhanced T1-weighted image demonstrates abnormal enhancement within the left sylvian fissure (arrow). There is also abnormal enhancement within the left lentiform nucleus (arrowhead). This is consistent with small infarction secondary to occlusion of penetrating vessels from the middle cerebral artery or focal encephalitis.

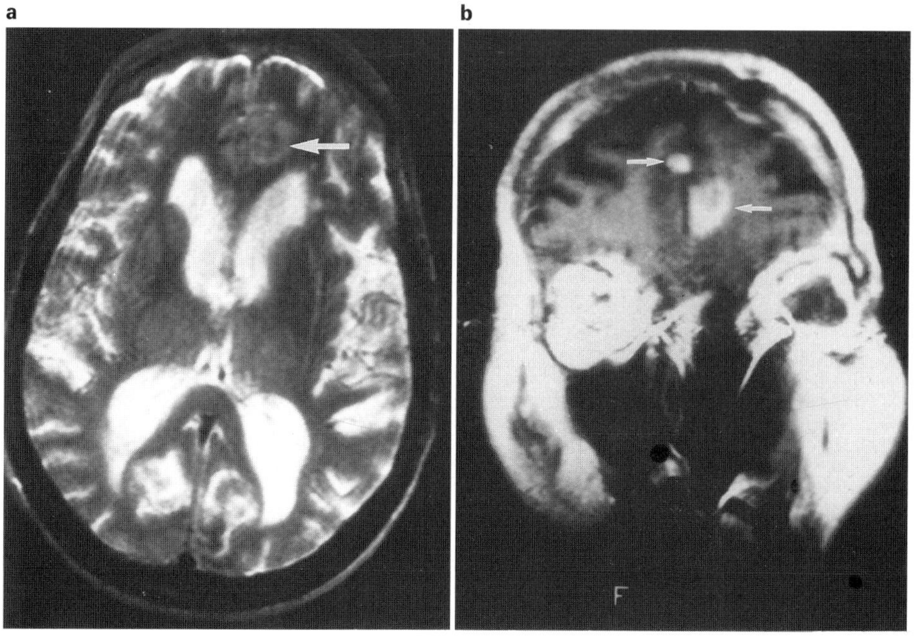

Fig. 14. Tuberculoma. Axial nonenhanced T2-weighted image (**a**) demonstrates a focal area of decreased signal intensity with a minimal rim of surrounding edema in the medial left frontal lobe (arrow). Following gadolinium administration, this coronal T1-weighted image (**b**) demonstrates enhancement of two parenchymal lesions (arrows). The sulcal and ventricular prominence was found to be secondary to infectious communicating hydrocephalus at autopsy.

lesions are small and without mass effect or significant edema. Some may show gadolinium enhancement. These lesions are not well delineated on CT.

Candida reaches the brain hematogenously from lung or gastrointestinal infections. The fungal form allows the agent to reach smaller arterioles resulting in small microabscesses. Small ring-enhancing or nodular-enhancing lesions may be seen on CT. Edema is typically minimal. With MRI examination, small hyperintense lesions are seen at the gray/white junction on T2-weighted images. With gadolinium administration small nodular- or ring-enhancing lesions can be seen.

Tuberculosis

Intracranial tuberculosis is seen more frequently, primarily related to the immunosuppressive states associated with AIDS infections. Most cases are secondary to hematogenous spread from pulmonary infections. Lesions can either be meningeal- or parenchymal-based.

Tuberculous meningitis causes a marked thickening of the meninges with a significant amount of purulent debris. This irritating debris frequently causes spasm or occlusion of small penetrating vessels resulting in infarction. This is particularly prominent in the ganglionic regions. CT scanning will frequently demonstrate increased density within the basal cisterns that enhances markedly following contrast administration. MRI also demonstrates abnormal signal intensity within the CSF of the basal cisterns. Marked meningeal and cisternal contrast enhancement is also a feature on MRI.

The hallmark of the parenchymal lesion is the tuberculoma. Multiple lesions are frequent. The lesions are round with a necrotic center. Edema is a variable manifestation. On CT, tuberculomas may be hypo- or hyperdense. Calcification is unusual, being seen in only 5% of cases. Most lesions will enhance following contrast administration. The lesion will appear ring-like, the central caseating material not enhancing. On MRI the caseating material is hypointense on the T1-weighted images and hyperintense on the T2-weighted images (fig. 14). The fibrous capsule is relatively isointense to the surrounding brain on T1-weighted images but is hypointense on T2-weighted images [19]. This results in a target appearance of the tuberculoma. With contrast administration there is typically ring enhancement of the lesion.

Cysticercosis

Cysticercosis is a disease caused by the parasite *Taenia solium.* The infection is related to the ingestion of undercooked pork. Between 60 and 90% of patients with cysticercosis develop CNS infection. Such an infection can either be parenchymal, meningeal or occur within the

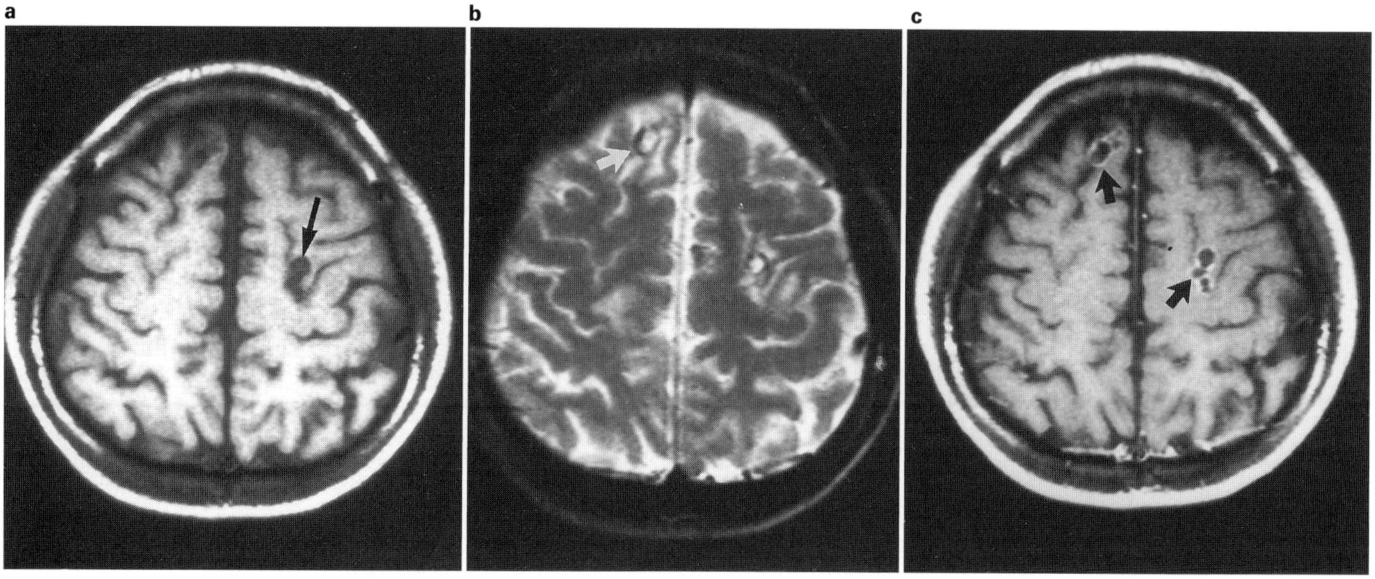

Fig. 15. Cysticercosis. Axial nonenhanced T1-weighted image (**a**) demonstrates an abnormal focus of decreased signal intensity in the left frontal parietal region (arrow). A T2-weighted image (**b**) at the same level demonstrates an inhomogeneous character of this lesion and a second lesion in the right frontal lobe (arrow). T1-weighted image following gadolinium (**c**) demonstrates irregular enhancement of the two lesions (arrows).

ventricular system. The parasitic embryo lodges within the brain or CSF developing a cystic covering and scolex. An intense inflammatory reaction surrounds the parenchymal infestation. A granulation and connective tissue capsule is then formed. This may be associated with decreasing edema and mass effect. Ultimately, the organism dies resulting in another significant inflammatory response and calcification. Symptoms include seizures, headache and dementia. Hydrocephalus may be seen secondary to meningeal infection or more commonly secondary to intraventricular cyst formation and obstruction.

In the acute setting, CT demonstrates multiple areas of low density. Nodular or ring enhancement may be seen. As the subacute state of infection begins, enhancement frequently lessens or disappears entirely. Late in the course of disease small calcifications are identified. Cysts may be identified on CT as low density lesions.

On MRI, areas of abnormal increased signal intensity are noted on T2-weighted images at the area of infestation [20]. Similar enhancement patterns are seen in MR as on CT. Cystic lesions are hypointense on T1-weighted images and hyperintense on T2-weighted images (fig. 15). Significant edema may be noted. Calcification is not well delineated on MR.

The density of the cyst material is nearly identical to that of CSF making the detection of intraventricular cysts difficult on CT scans. The high protein content within the cyst gives it a slightly hyperintense appearance, with respect to normal CSF, on T1-weighted and proton density-weighted MR images. This allows improved detection of intraventricular lesions by MR. The lesions are frequently isointense to CSF on T2-weighted images.

Lyme Disease

Lyme disease is an infection caused by a spirochete, *Borrelia burgdorferi.* The spirochete is transmitted by a tick and is endemic in the Northeast. There is typically a skin rash which develops early in the illness. The rash may disappear before neurologic symptoms begin. Most cases with neurologic involvement will resolve, even without treatment, but some fatalities have been reported. The patients frequently present with meningitis-type symptoms or cranial and peripheral neuropathies. The gross pathologic appearance is similar to multiple sclerosis. CT scanning is relatively insensitive for the disease. If the study is abnormal, vague low density will be seen within the white matter. MRI typically shows multiple foci of abnormal increased signal intensity within the deep white

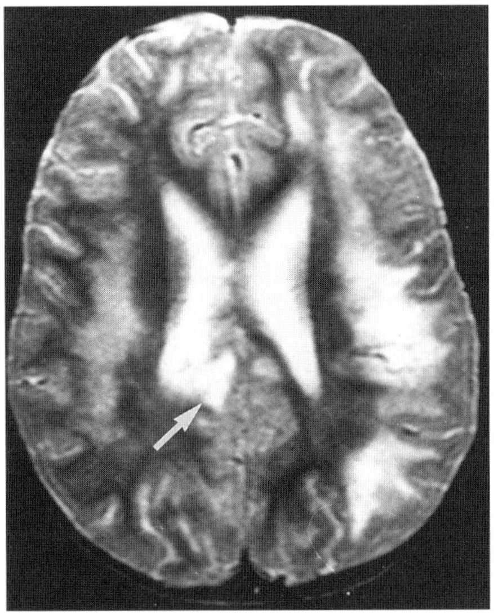

Fig. 16. Lyme disease. Axial T2-weighted image at the level of the body of the lateral ventricles demonstrates marked subcortical and deep white matter-increased signal. There is also an abnormal signal within the corpus callosum (arrow).

matter on T2-weighted images (fig. 16). Usually the lesions are small and relatively well circumscribed, but occasionally the lesions may be more prominent and confluent [21]. Resolution of the abnormalities has been reported with appropriate treatment.

Acquired Immunodeficiency Syndrome

It is estimated that between 400,000 and 500,000 individuals will have AIDS by 1994 and that 2–4 million will be HIV-positive. Approximately 10% of patients with AIDS present with neurologic symptoms, while approximately 60% of patients will have neurologic symptoms during the course of their illness.

The neuroradiologic manifestations of AIDS include meningoependymal disease, cerebral atrophy, mass lesions and white matter disease [22].

Meningoependymal disease is most commonly secondary to cryptococcal infection. Other agents, such as tuberculosis, can also be associated with meningoependymal disease in the AIDS patient.

The most common abnormality of the brain seen in AIDS patients is cerebral atrophy. This appears secondary to HIV cerebritis, an infection primarily involving the neurons. It is usually associated with the AIDS dementia complex. Abnormal ventricular and sulcal prominence is seen on CT and MR. Typically the signal intensity on both CT and MR is normal. No abnormal enhancement is identified.

Although a wide variety of pathogens may cause mass lesions within the brain, toxoplasmosis and lymphoma remain the most common. Toxoplasmosis is a protozoan. It can be seen as a congenital infection giving a similar neuroradiologic appearance as cytomegalovirus, including subependymal and parenchymal calcifications. In those cases associated with AIDS, the lesions present as focal masses. The lesions may be single or multiple. They may be hemorrhagic. On plain CT the lesions are frequently hypodense without contrast and significant edema may be present. With intravenous contrast administration, nodular or ring-enhancing lesions may be seen. On MRI the lesions are typically hypointense on T1- and hyperintense on T2-weighted images. If hemorrhagic, the lesions will demonstrate signal intensity consistent with the state of the hemorrhagic products (fig. 17). Nodular or ring enhancement is seen following gadolinium administration.

AIDS-related lymphoma can have an identical appearance with toxoplasmosis. As opposed to primary lymphoma, AIDS-related lymphoma is not typically seen in the immediate periventricular area. There is a slight propensity for lymphoma to be seen in the basal ganglia and to be somewhat larger, on average, than toxoplasmosis. Nodular or ring enhancement is seen with contrast administration. On MRI the lesions may be relatively hypointense on T2-weighted images. This may be secondary to the hypercellularity and high nuclear/cytoplasmic ratio in these tumors. Extensive edema is also a feature of lymphoma. Enhancement with gadolinium may be nodular or ring enhancing. Both toxoplasmosis and lymphomatous lesions can exist within the same individual. A recent MR study of over 300 patients with AIDS demonstrated that patients with mass lesions were the only group whose diagnostic study significantly benefitted from contrast administration [23]. This has significant implications relating to imaging time, contrast costs and personnel needle-stick risk.

The most common white matter lesion without mass effect in AIDS patients is HIV cerebritis or encephalopathy. Typically such lesions are manifest by bilateral, symmetric abnormal increased signal intensity on T2-weighted MR images. The lesions have a predominate periventricular and deep white matter location. The finding may or may not be associated with concomitant cerebral atrophy. The lesions are difficult to detect on CT. These lesions do not show contrast enhancement.

a b c

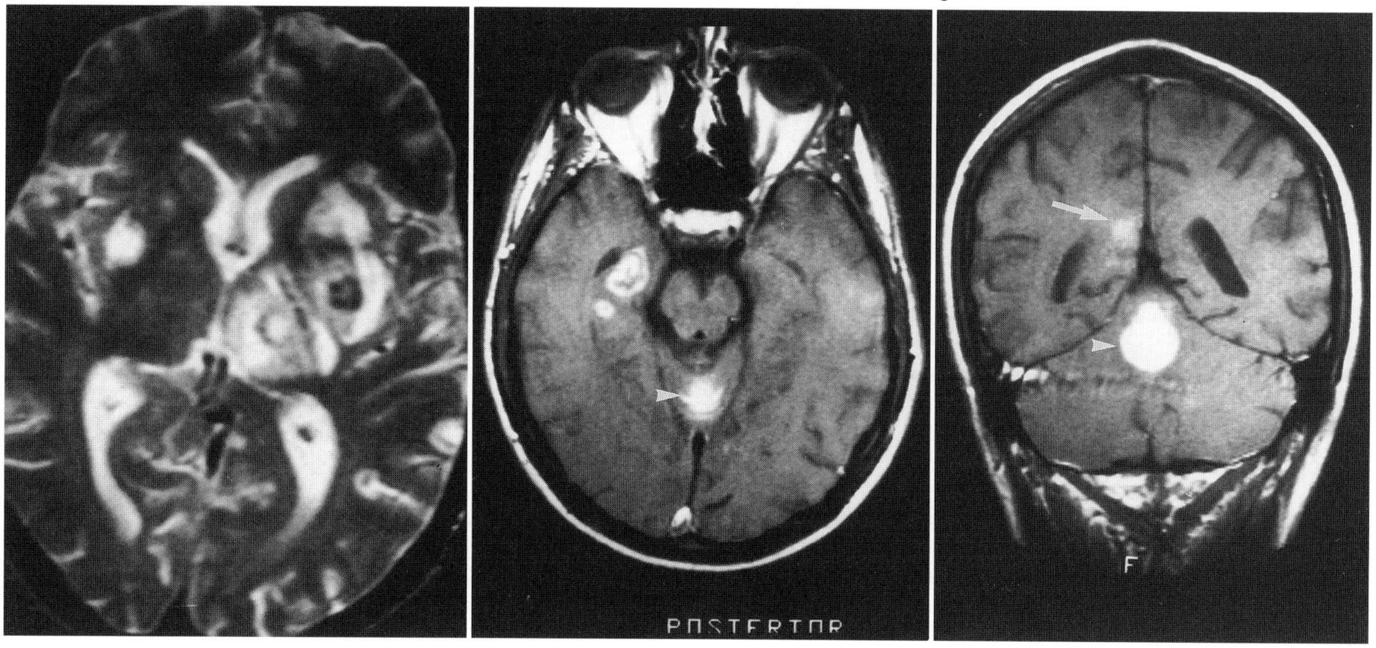

Fig. 17a–c. Toxoplasmosis, AIDS-related. Axial T2-weighted image (**a**) demonstrates multiple foci of abnormal increased signal intensity. Lesions within the left putamen and left thalamus are partially hemorrhagic as evidenced by their decreased signal intensity, consistent with deoxyhemoglobin. In a second patient with toxoplasmosis, axial and coronal gadolinium-enhanced T1-weighted images demonstrate multiple areas of abnormal enhancement. The two lesions within the right temporal lobe were found to represent toxoplasmosis. The medial right occipital lesion (arrow) was also found to represent toxoplasmosis. The large vermian lesion (arrowheads) was found to represent lymphoma at autopsy.

a b

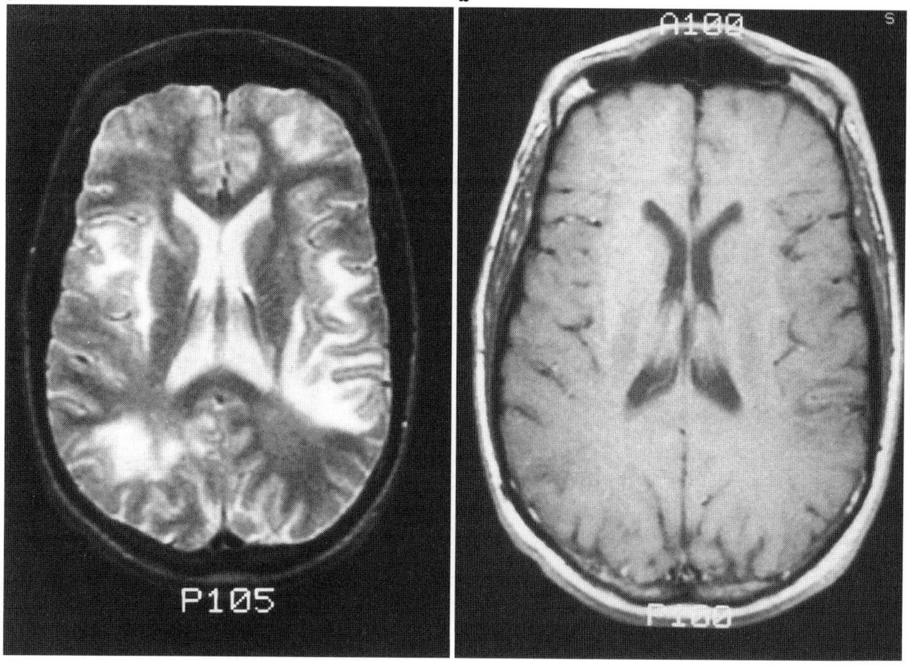

Fig. 18. AIDS-related progressive multifocal leukoencephalopathy. Axial T2-weighted image (**a**) demonstrates abnormal increased signal intensity within the subcortical regions bilaterally. Other small scattered foci are seen throughout the deep white matter. No significant mass effect is seen. Mild atrophy is noted. The T1-weighted image following gadolinium (**b**) demonstrates low signal intensity in the region of the larger lesions. No abnormal enhancement is seen.

The other significant disease associated with white matter lesions without mass effect in AIDS patients is progressive multifocal leukoencephalopathy. This entity is associated with immunosuppressed states and is secondary to infection with a papova virus. The virus produces demyelination and necrosis of the white matter. Death typically ensues within several months after diagnosis. On CT the lesion demonstrates decreased attenuation in the peripheral white matter. There is usually no mass effect or abnormal enhancement. The lesion is best detected on T2-weighted MR images (fig. 18). The lesions are hyperintense and without mass effect [24]. There is relative periventricular sparing. The lesions are typically bilateral but may not be symmetric. The parietal lobes appear to be the most commonly affected. Enhancement on MR is unusual.

Conclusions

A wide variety of infections within the brain can now be imaged. Although CT may be useful for detecting calcifications associated with some lesions, MRI is the prime modality in the evaluation of intracranial infection. In most circumstances contrast administration will be necessary. Imaging studies will continue to be useful, not only in the diagnosis of intracranial infection but also in the evaluation of therapeutic efficacy.

Acknowledgements

The author would like to thank Barbara Smith for her help in the preparation of this manuscript.

References

1 Brant-Zawadzki M, Davis PL, Crooks LE, et al: NMR demonstration of cerebral abnormalities: Comparison with CT. AJNR 1983;4:117–124.

2 Chang KH, Han MH, Roh JK, Kim IO, Han MC, Kim CW: Gd-DTPA-enhanced MR imaging of the brain in patients with meningitis: Comparison with CT. AJNR 1990;11:69–76.

3 Zimmerman RA, Patel S, Bilaniuk L: Demonstration of purulent bacterial intracranial infections by computed tomography. AJR 1976; 127:155–165.

4 Mathews VP, Smith RR, Bognanno JR, Kuharik MA, Edwards MK, Harris TM: Gd-DTPA enhanced MR of meningitis: Initial clinical experience (abstract). AJNR 1989;10: 1290.

5 Rabe EF: Subdural effusions in infants. Pediatr Clin North Am 1967;14:831–850.

6 Weingarten K, Zimmerman RD, Becker RD, Heier LA, Haimes AB, Deck MDF: Subdural and epidural empyemas: MR imaging. AJNR 1989;10:81–87.

7 Crain MR, Yuh WTC, Greene GM, et al: Cerebral ischemia: Evaluation with contrast-enhanced MR imaging. AJNR 1991;12:631–639.

8 Harris TM, Smith RR, Koch KJ: Gadolinium-DTPA enhanced MR imaging of septic dural sinus thrombosis. J Comput Assist Tomogr 1989;13:682–684.

9 Mathews VP, Smith RR: Infections of the lateral choroid plexus. AJNR, in press.

10 Enzmann DR, Britt RH, Yeager AS: Experimental brain abscess evolution: Computed tomographic and neuropathologic correlation. Radiology 1979;133:113–122.

11 Haimes AB, Zimmerman RD, Morgello S, Weingarten K, Becker RD, Jennis R, Deck MDF: MR imaging of brain abscesses. AJNR 1989;10:279–291.

12 Goldberg HI, Titelbaum DS, Grossman RI, Hackney DB, Filaniuk LT, Zimmerman RA: High field MR of brain abscess (abstract). AJNR 1988;9:1036.

13 Neils EW, Lukin R, Tomsick TA, Tew JM: Magnetic resonance imaging and computerized tomography scanning of herpes simplex encephalitis. J Neurosurg 1987;67:592–594.

14 Jungreis CA, Grossman RI: Intracranial infections and inflammatory diseases; in Latchaw RE (ed): MR and CT Imaging of the Head, Neck and Spine. St Louis, Mosby-Year Book, 1991, pp 303–346.

15 Gomori JM, Grossman RI, Goldberg HI, Zimmerman RA, Bilaniuk LT: Intracranial hematomas: Imaging by high-field MR. Radiology 1985;157:87–93.

16 Atlas SW, Grossman RI, Goldberg HI, Hackney DB, Bilaniuk LT, Zimmerman RA: MR diagnosis of acute disseminated encephalomyelitis. J Comput Assist Tomogr 1986;10: 798–801.

17 Caldemeyer KS, Harris TM, Smith RR, Edwards MK: Gadolinium enhancement in acute disseminated encephalomyelitis. J Comput Assist Tomogr 1991;15:673–675.

18 Smith RR, Kuharik MA: Inflammation and infection of the brain; in Cohen MD, Edwards MD (eds): Magnetic Resonance Imaging of Children. Philadelphia, Decker, 1990, pp 221–275.

19 Gupta RK, Jena A, Sharma A, Guha DK, Khushu S, Gupta AK: MR imaging of intracranial tuberculomas. J Comput Assist Tomogr 1988; 12:280–285.

20 Zee C-S, Segall HD, Boswell W, Ahmadi J, Nelson M, Colletti P: MR imaging of neurocysticercosis. J Comput Assist Tomogr 1988;12: 927–934.

21 Fernandez RE, Rothberg M, Ferencz G, Wujak D: Lyme disease of the CNS: MR imaging findings in 14 cases. AJNR 1990;11:479–481.

22 Levy R, Rosenbloom S, Perrett LV: Neuroradiologic findings in AIDS: A review of 200 cases. AJNR 1986;7:833–839.

23 Gean-Marton AD, Eisenberg AD, Kirsch CFE, Demas BE, Norman D: The utility of gadolinium administration in the evaluation of HIV-positive patients with suspected CNS pathology. American Society of Neuroradiology Annual Meeting, Washington, 1991.

24 Hansman Whiteman ML, Post MJ, Berger J, Tate LG, Bruce J, Limonte LP: PML in 45 HIV-positive patients: Neuroimaging with pathologic correlation. Radiological Society of North America Annual Meeting, Chicago, 1991.

Pediatr Neurosurg 1992;18:105–116

Hiroshi Otsubo
Sylvester H. Chuang
Paul A. Hwang
David Gilday
Harold J. Hoffman

Department of Neurology, Diagnostic Imaging, Neurosurgery, The Hospital for Sick Children and University of Toronto, Toronto, Canada

Neuroimaging for Investigation of Seizures in Children

Key Words
Seizures
Epilepsy
Neuroimaging

Abstract
In patients with structural abnormalities of the brain with poor seizure control by medication, epilepsy surgery becomes a very important tool for seizure control. Numerous radiological imaging studies are being used for studying the abnormality in order to aid in the planning of surgery. Included in the radiological imaging modalities are CT, MR, and Xenon CT, SPECT and PET. In future, perfusion and diffusion MR as well as MEG mapping will become part of the investigative tool. The following paper is a summary and discussion of the usefulness of different modalities in different disease entities with a proposal for the method of investigation.

Introduction

The Classification of Seizures
The international classification of epileptic seizures was proposed in 1981; (1) partial seizures including simple partial seizures, complex partial seizures, and partial seizures evolving to secondarily generalized seizures (tonic-clonic, tonic, or clonic), (2) generalized seizures (convulsive or nonconvulsive), and (3) unclassified epileptic seizures [17]. In 1989, an international classification of epilepsies and epileptic syndrome has been proposed, because of the necessity of a classification of syndromes rather than diseases [18]. It separated localization-related epilepsies from generalized epilepsies. The localization-related epilepsies were divided to idiopathic and symptomatic including temporal lobe epilepsy, frontal, parietal and occipital, and cryptogenic.

Neuroimaging Studies for Seizures
A number of imaging techniques are available to complement electrophysiological methods when evaluating patients with intractable localization-related epilepsies and epileptic syndromes prior to possible surgical treatment. These techniques assess structural as well as functional abnormalities. Previously, computed tomography (CT) was used as the main tool to look for structural abnormalities in the evaluation of patients with epilepsy [94, 28].

Recently, magnetic resonance imaging (MRI) has proven to be better in the detection of small epileptogenic lesions, especially hippocampal sclerosis that corresponds to temporal lobe epilepsy [13, 39, 55, 60, 76]. In functional imaging, positron emission tomography (PET) has been used to identify the epileptogenic area both with perfusion and metabolic studies [15, 48, 85]. Localized epi-

Dr. Sylvester H. Chuang
Department of Diagnostic Imaging
The Hospital for Sick Children
555 University Avenue
Toronto, Ont. M5G 1X8 (Canada)

leptiform discharges that correspond to abnormal regional cerebral blood flow (rCBF) are also demonstrated by single photon emission computed tomography (SPECT) using ^{99m}Tc-hexamethylpropylenamine oxime (HMPAO), interictally and postictally [36, 79, 80]. This review of neuroimaging studies for epilepsies and epileptic syndromes in children is discussed in terms of partial seizures (focal or local) and partial seizures evolving into generalized seizures, which were most likely symptomatic localization-related epilepsies and epileptic syndromes. In addition, infantile spasms (West syndrome) which was classified in generalized epilepsies is highlighted by current functional neuroimaging studies. Conventional CT and xenon-inhalated CT, MRI, SPECT using ^{99m}Tc HMPAO and PET will be reviewed in this article.

Modalities of Neuroimaging Study for Epilepsy in Children

Computed Tomography

In the investigation in epilepsy children, pre- and post-contrast-enhanced CT scans are routinely performed. In the cases in which temporal lobe epilepsy is suspected, scans are performed with 5 mm thickness in the plane of the temporal lobe, i.e. −5 to −10 degree to the baseline. Coronal views of the temporal lobes are also obtained after contrast enhancement.

Xenon CT

Inhalation xenon CT is not performed routinely except for suspected perfusion problem or unexplained temporal lobe seizures. Routine CT scans are always performed prior to Xenon CT examination. Selected slices for the xenon study are planned before patient inhalation of xenon gas is started. Only a maximum of 3 slices are allowed per examination and therefore the choice of location becomes extremely important. Scans were repeated at the same level at different stages of inhalation and computer calculations were made at the end for the xenon gas distribution. This required knowledge of the patient's hemoglobin and CO_2.

Magnetic Resonance Imaging

The routine sequence for the investigation of temporal lobe epilepsy by MRI consists of T1 sagittal localizer scan, T2 coronal and T2 axial scans. The T2 scans performed in 2 planes are such that small signal intensity changes in the temporal lobes will not be missed, ensuring that false positive and negative results are eliminated.

In children under 2 years of age, heavily weighted T2 images are performed with a TR of 2800 and a TE of 135 because the brain is not fully myelinated. Matrix size varies between 192 and 256. Motion and pulsation artifacts are compensated for. Gadolinium diethylenetriamine pentaacetic acid (Gd-DTPA) is not routinely used unless a tumor is suspected.

Single Photon Emission Computed Tomography

SPECT was performed with ^{99m}Tc-HMPAO in order to study the rCBF during the interictal period and immediately postictally, within 10 min after seizure onset, within the epilepsy monitoring unit. An intravenous line was placed, the patient was kept in a quiet room with dim light and the ears plugged, and then injected intravenously with 14 mCi (520 mBq) of ^{99m}Tc-HMPAO. Twenty minutes later, tomographic acquisitions were begun using a single rotating head camera equipped with a high resolution collimator. Data were processed for 128 × 128 matrices, with 128 projections of 20 s each using an elliptical orbit over 360°. Following uniformity corrections for each projection, 1.2-cm slice thickness transaxials were reconstructed using filtered back projection with a Hanning filter (frequency cutoff = 1.0 cycles/cm).

Positron Emission Tomography

PET is not routinely used for investigation of the children with intractable seizures. For the patient who has no structural abnormality on either CT or MRI, PET is used to confirm the finding of at functional abnormality on SPECT. We study patients with fluorine-18 labeled fluorodeoxyglucose (18-FDG) to determine the local cerebral metabolic rate in the utilization of glucose (LCMRglc). The tomograph at the McMaster University has a spatial resolution of 8 mm (full width at half maximum) in the plane, and a slice thickness of 12 mm, capable of resolving voxels of less than 1 cm^3. Sixteen overlapping slices of the brain are examined sequentially, obtained in a plane of 5° above the orbitomeatal line, from the hippocampal gyrus to the vertex. The entire examination lasts less than 1 h, during which the patient is sedated.

Neuroimaging Studies for Epilepsy Surgery

The incidence of patients with epilepsy in the general population is reported to be from 0.5 to 0.6% [11, 63]. In this group patients with refractory seizures range between 20 and 40%, approximately 30% of whom have intractable partial epilepsies. In terms of epilepsy surgery, the sur-

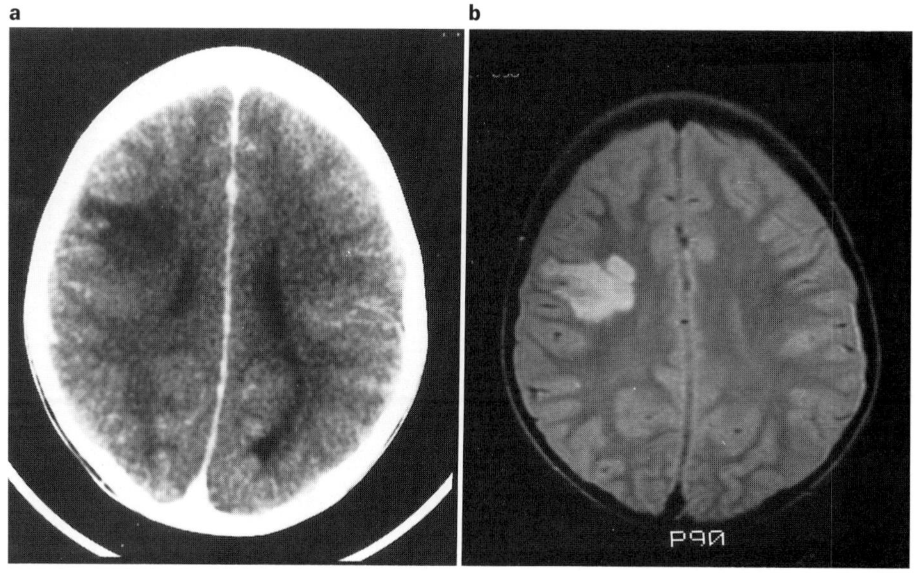

Fig. 1. Focal cortical dysplasia. A 5-year-old boy with left partial motor seizure, contrast CT showing low attenuation area over right frontal central regions, without any contrast enhancement (**a**). Proton density MR shows high signal intensity lesion over between the gray and white matter on the right frontal central regions (**b**).

gical candidates constitute 10–25% of the patients with the complex partial seizures [33, 56].

In our institution, CT has been used since 1976, SPECT since 1987 and MRI since 1988, for the detection of the seizure foci in pediatric patients who were monitored with scalp electroencephalogram (EEG), special EEG and closed circuit video telemetry on the epilepsy monitoring unit. Of the patients with resectable epileptogenic focus (surgical candidates), there were 80 children between 1987 and 1990. Forty of them had temporal lobectomy, extratemporal focal cortical excision or hemidecortication, under electrocorticogram.

In the 40 patients with epilepsy surgery, preoperative neuroimaging studies of 37 patients were reviewed to correlate between abnormal findings on imaging studies and the pathology of epileptogenic lesion in the temporal and extratemporal regions (excluding hemimegalencephaly). All 37 patients had abnormal EEG findings on the epilepsy monitoring unit, including 30 patients presenting ictal and interictal epileptogenic foci. Twenty-seven of 32 patients had MRI-demonstrated abnormalities which corresponded to the epileptogenic focus. Of 28 patients with interictal and postictal SPECT study, focal and regional abnormalities correlating to the epileptogenic area were detected in 21. Of the 37 patients who were examined with CT scan, 23 had lesions in the localized epileptogenic region. Neoplasms in 13 patients were detected with nonenhanced and/or enhanced CT. Of the MRI, SPECT and CT studies, MRI and SPECT had a higher ratio of correlated abnormality to the epileptogenic focus than CT, namely 84 and 75 in comparison to 62%.

Specific Neuroimaging of Typical Epilepsies and Epileptic Syndromes

Focal Cortical Dysplasia

Focal cortical dysplasia, due to neuronal migration disorders, is characterized by disorganization of cortical architecture, with aberrant columnar and laminar neuronal arrangement [6, 27]. The neuronal microdysgenesis in patients with partial seizures were reported, associated with localized, not infrequently widespread, epileptogenic area on EEG [64, 65, 84].

Abnormal gyral formation was found on CT in 1 patient out of our 9 patients with pathologically confirmed focal cortical dysplasia. Increased attenuation with negative enhancement was detected in 1 patient, a low attenuation area in 2. Five of 9 patients had no abnormal findings on CT. MRI demonstrated abnormalities in 8 of 9 patients with typical findings of focal cortical dysplasia in 6. Two patietns had increased intensity signal on T2 imaging but not typical findings of focal cortical dysplasia (fig. 1). One patient had no abnormal findings on MRI. Interictal SPECT detected decreased rCBF in 7 of 8 patients, postictal SPECT demonstrated increased rCBF in the same epileptogenic focus in 2. One patient had hypometabolism on PET over the same region as decreased rCBF on SPECT.

MRI is superior to CT for detection of the cortical and subcortical derangements of severe dysplastic lesions, mild to moderate dysplasia which are more subtle lesions are better seen on MRI, whereas CT findings are normal [46]. Anatomical extent of the epileptogenic area was

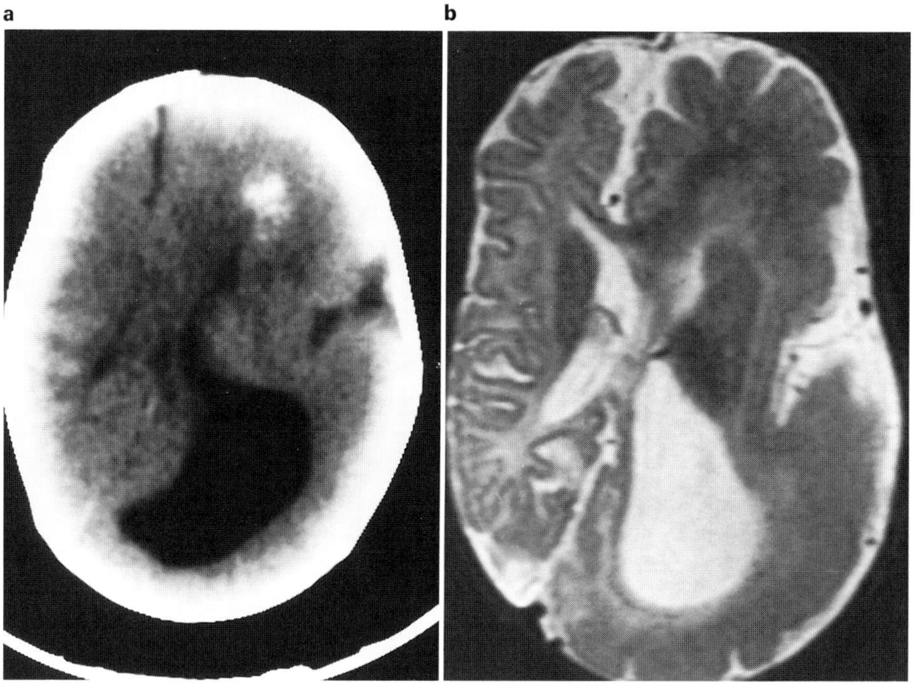

Fig. 2. Hemimegalencephaly. A 4-month-old girl with intractable seizures consisting of partial motor and secondary generalized seizures as well as infantile spasms; CT shows remarkable left hemispheric and ventricular enlargement (**a**). MRI better demonstrates abnormal gyral formation over the left hemisphere and loss of gray and white matter differentiation (**b**).

larger than can be detected on CT and MRI. This discrepancy is considered to be spread of epileptogenic foci, secondary epileptogenesis, or widespread migrational abnormality not identified by structural imaging studies [64]. Since functional imaging studies have been established to detect epileptogenic foci, perfusion and metabolic disturbance in the regions of neuronal migration disorders are well demonstrated on SPECT and PET.

Hemimegalencephaly

Hemimegalencephaly results in a hypertrophied, malformed hemisphere with marked histologic disorganization [9, 20, 49, 52, 71, 88]. The patients with hemimegalencephaly present with a triad of clinical findings including intractable seizures, developmental delay and progressive hemiparesis [4, 43, 44, 57]. Neurophysiological studies show a lateralized disorganized background activity with multifocal epileptiform activities in the involved hemisphere, and modified hypsarrhythmia [32, 86].

CT scan in 11 patients with hemimegalencephaly showed hemispheric hypertrophy in all patients and were associated with significant ipsilateral lateral ventricular dilation in 10. MRI defined abnormal gyration and gray-white matter differentiation more precisely than CT [86]. SPECT showed localization-increased rCBF over the epileptogenic area between interictal and postictal, instead of diffuse decreased rCBF over involved hemisphere (fig. 2).

Hemospheric hypertrophy and ipsilateral lateral ventricular enlargement are well defined on CT [25]. However, poorly differentiated gray and white matter with increased cortical thickness and abnormal gyration with appearance similar to pachygyria are better demonstrated on MRI than newer generation CT [4, 43].

Tuberous Sclerosis

Typical clinical triad of tuberous sclerosis is well known as consisting of sebacous adenomas, mental deficiency and epilepsy [10, 91]. Seizures begin early in childhood, even as infantile spasms.

Hamartomas area seen as increased signal intensity on T2-weighted images on MRI. They are seen over the epileptogenic region (fig. 3). Subependymal calcifications on CT do not correspond to seizure focus.

Subependymal nodules are commonly seen as calcified lesions; therefore CT is most sensitive in detecting them [26]. Calcifications may occur in the cortex or at the gray-white matter interface with or without hamartoma but are much rarer. The cortical tubers, which occur at the gray-white matter junction and in the cortex itself, are better demonstrated on MRI [58] and correlate better with EEG abnormalities. Contrast enhancement in these patients in the subependymal nodules in the region of the foramen of Monro on CT usually indicates degeneration to giant cell tumor. Though similar findings are seen in MRI with Gd-DTPA, it is much more sensitive and regular enhance-

a b

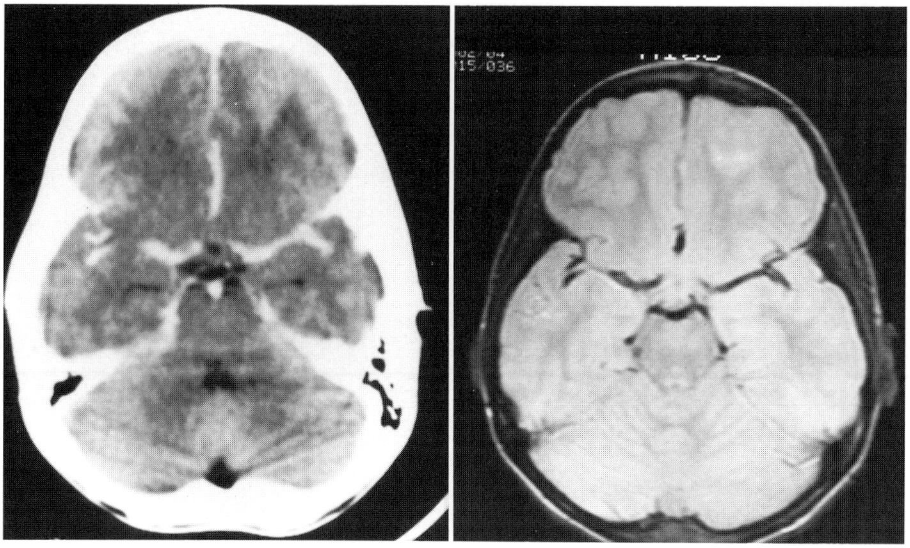

Fig. 3. Tuberous sclerosis. A 10-year-old girl presented with signs of tuberous sclerosis and complex partial seizures with secondarily generalized epilepsy; contrast-enhanced CT shows low attenuation area over left inferior frontal region (**a**). Proton density MRI shows a high intensity signal area and loss of gray and white matter differentiation over the left frontal lobe (**b**).

ment of tissues in and around the tuber are seen in some cases. Functional imaging studies are helpful in order to define the epileptogenic focus, but calcified lesions which cause decreased rCBF or hypometabolism are a problem in localizing the corresponding epileptogenic focus.

Sturge-Weber Syndrome

Sturge [81] described a patient with facial nevus flammeus and cerebral malformation in 1879, followed by Weber [92] who identified the characteristic calcification seen on x-ray in 1922, so that this syndrome then became known as the Sturge-Weber syndrome. The clinical course of this disease varies; if seizures begin in the 1st month of life, there appears to be a high risk of progressive mental deterioration with severe hemiplegia and intractable seizures. In our institution, pediatric patients with the Sturge-Weber syndrome associated with early infantile onset intractable seizures consisting of partial motor seizures or partial seizures secondarily generalized undergo early unilateral hemispherectomy of the involved hemisphere [59, 72]. In the other type of childhood onset, lesions restricted to parietal and occipital lobes produce slightly milder but still intractable seizures in childhood [51].

Of the 29 patients that had CT, 18 showed diffuse hemispheric involvement with atrophic change. Intracranial calcifications were detected in 17 patients, and were first demonstrated as early as 3 weeks. Ten had hemispheric calcifications involving two or more lobes, while the other 7 patients had frontal, parietal and occipital calcifications on CT [59, 72]. Our recent MRI findings in 3 patients with the childhood onset type of the Sturge-Weber syndrome showed calcifications in parietooccipital regions in 2 patients, occipital demyelination and calcification in 1. SPECT demonstrated regional increased rCBF over parietal and posterior temporal lobes in 2 patients, and multifocal increased rCBF in 1 (fig. 4).

CT shows gyriform intracranial calcification in the watershed regions, progressive atrophy and loss of volume of the affected hemisphere in the infant onset form. In the localized form, the vascular enhancement is mostly in the parietooccipital region, often involving the posterior temporal region as well. Choroid plexus in the affected hemisphere is usually involved and shows increased attenuation with contrast. MRI may show vascular enhancement with Gd-DTPA, but does not show watershed calcifications as well as CT does. Functional imaging studies with Xe CT and SPECT demonstrate varied rCBF, increased rCBF is considered to represent increased flow through the pial angiomatosis; on the other hand, decreased rCBF shows the secondary underlying brain ischemia which correlates with the calcified area of the interictal localization-related epileptogenic focus. Despite the fact that MRI does not demonstrate calcification as well as CT, it shows angiomatous enhancement better than CT.

Tumors

In localization-related epilepsy, partial seizures are common evidence of mass lesions; particularly these lesions locate in temporal lobe [70]. The majority of tumors producing seizures especially in temporal lobe are

a b c

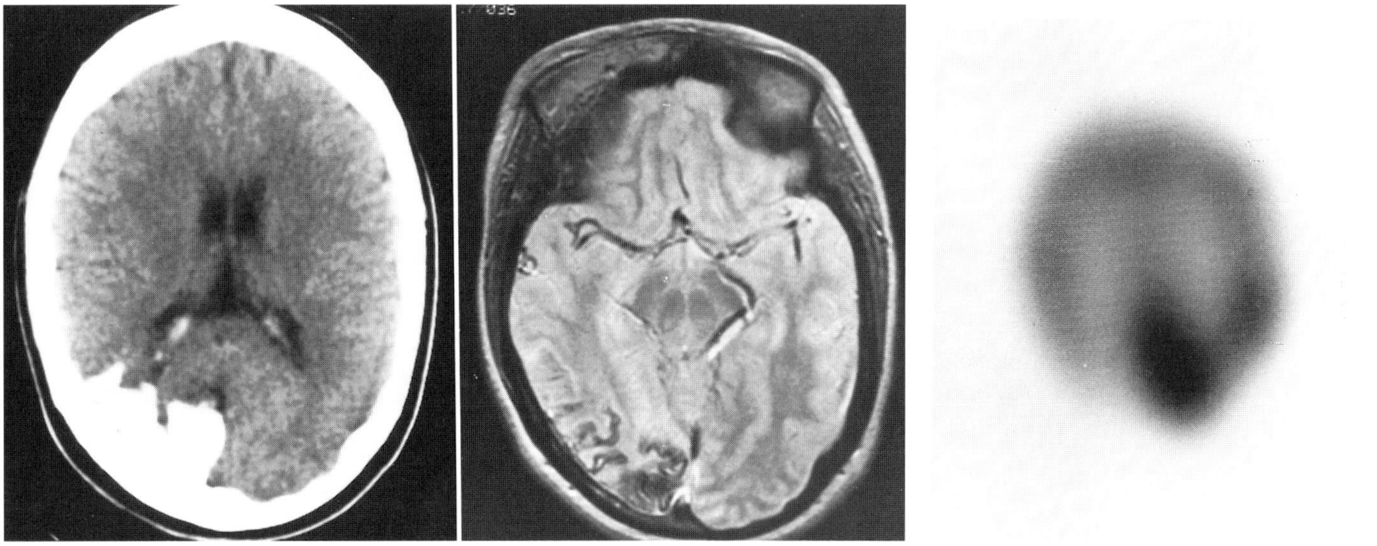

Fig. 4. Sturge-Weber syndrome. A 14-year-old girl with left facial nevus and intractable complex partial seizures shows calcification in the right occipital and posterior temporal lobes on CT (**a**). T_2W MRI shows the right occipital demyelination and gyriform calcification (**b**). Interictal SPECT detected decreased rCBF on the right occipital lobe (**c**).

benign, long-standing neoplasms, so that many of these patients have had a long history of intractable complex partial seizures [22]. One third of temporal lobectomy in children are pathologically diagnosed benign tumors such as low grade astrocytoma, oligodendroglioma, ganglioglioma, hamartoma, mixed glioma. Ganglioglioma are most representative of long-standing tumors in temporal lobe [62]. Pathologically ganglioglioma is a mixture of neuronal components and astrocytic elements [29]. Follow-up prognosis in the patients with mass lesion after temporal lobectomy are reported as better than those without mass lesions. The anterior temporal lobectomy should extend the cortical excision on the basis of epileptiform activity detected by electrocorticography [22].

In patients with ganglioglioma, cystic components appeared as low attenuation area in 4 out of 9 patients. T2-weighted MRI showed increased signal intensity in 5 out of 6 patients; contrast enhancement with Gd-DTPA was seen on T1-weighted MRI in all gangliogliomas prior to surgery. One lesion which only had small calcification on CT was missed on MRI (fig. 5) [62].

In one sense, on CT scan, over 90% of temporal lobe gliomas were found to have little enhancement, no mass effect, calcification or cystic components. In another sense, enhancement with contrast materials was seen in about one half of cases [21].

Mesial Temporal Sclerosis

Mesial temporal sclerosis (MTS), hippocampal sclerosis, has been recognized as the most common symptomatic pathology, and maybe associated with other pathological lesions, in patients with temporal lobe epilepsy [3, 24, 30, 31, 50, 53, 74]. Although the pathophysiologic mechanism of MTS has not been established, localized anoxic infarction [66], serious childhood illness [24] and serious seizures at an early age [3, 14] have been proposed as the cause of neuronal damage in the hippocampus. The incidence of dual pathology with a significant coexistent MTS and extrahippocampal pathologies varies from 8 to 22% [3].

In our series, MTS in pediatric patients are mostly associated with ipsilateral temporal lobe tumors as well as congenital abnormalities, namely 7 out of 12 patients. Asymmetry of temporal lobe and high signal intensity on T2-weighted imaging in mesial temporal region are seen on MR scans in patients with isolated MTS, patients who have normal findings on CT scan (fig. 6). SPECT shows decreased focal and regional CBF in the inferomedial temporal regions interictally.

Prior to the MRI era, the ability to determine focal atrophic change of the temporal lobes by CT, with intravenous contrast and/or intrathecal enhancement, was found not to be reliable [28, 94]. Although accuracy of MRI findings in MTS are controversial, specific findings

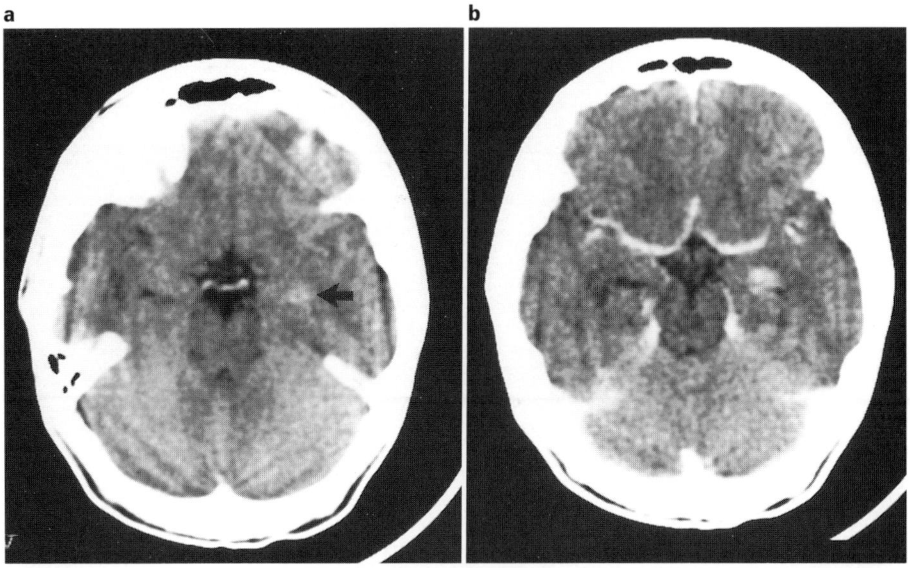

Fig. 5. Ganglioglioma. A 15-year-old boy with intractable complex partial seizures; CT shows small calcification in left medial temporal region (**a**, arrow), which was missed on non-Gd MRI. Contrast CT shows the calcified mass with some enhancement (**b**).

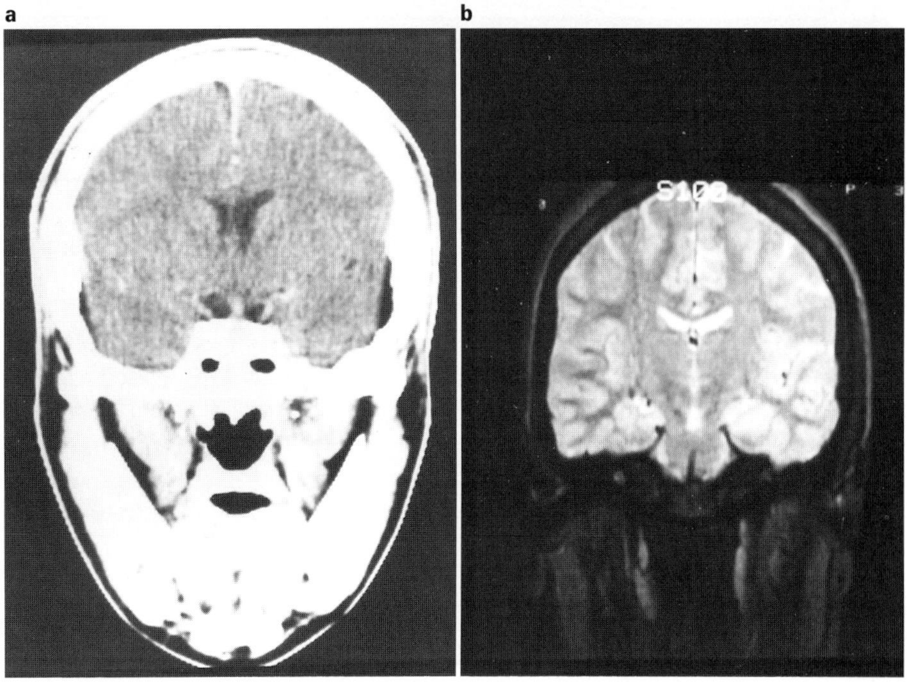

Fig. 6. Mesial temporal sclerosis. A 16-year-old girl with a 10-year history of complex partial seizures; no remarkable abnormality is found on contrasted coronal CT (**a**). Coronal T_2W MRI shows high intensity signal over the left inferior mesial temporal lobe (**b**).

such as increased T2 signal, reduction of hippocampal volume, 'verticalization' of sylvian fissure, and loss of gray-white matter differentiation in the temporal lobe are more accurate than CT scans [2, 12, 31, 45, 78]. The accuracy of MRI scans varies greatly in different reports though the ones with low false negative results tend to have high false positive results. In the patients with temporal lobe epilepsy, PET has been reported as being particularly sensitive, more so than SPECT in showing lateralization of the lesions [79].

Rasmussen Syndrome

A syndrome of chronic encephalitis with intractable focal epilepsy was described in 1958 by Rasmussen [68]. The patients presented with severe focal epilepsy, epilepsia partialis continua, associated with slowly progressive neurologic deterioration and progressive lateralized brain destruction. The surgical tissues microscopically revealed encephalitis with widespread perivascular cuffs of round cells and scattered microglial nodules [1, 34, 69].

Our previous series reported that CT showed 3 hemiatrophies, 2 focal atrophies and 1 normal finding in 6

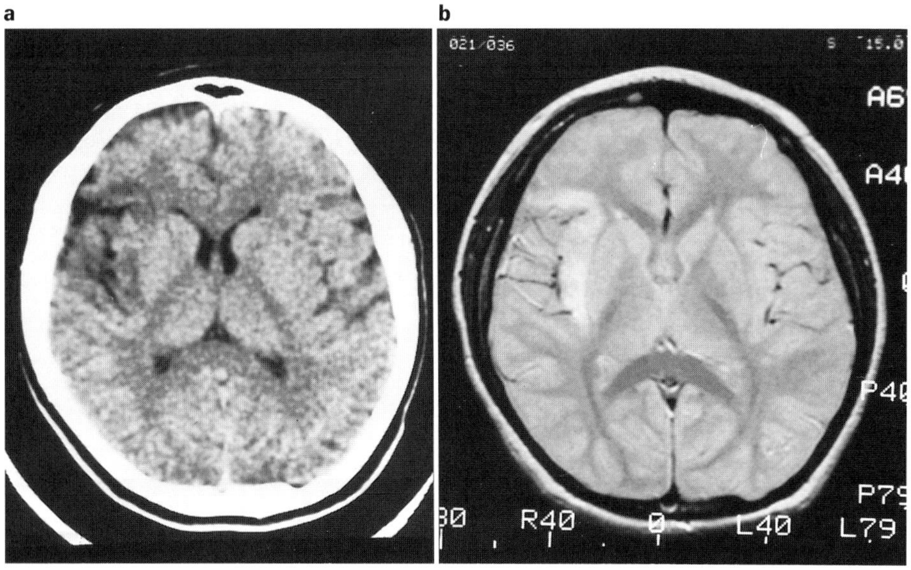

Fig. 7. Rasmussen syndrome. An 11-year-old boy was presented with epilepsia partialis continua, progressive left hemiparesis and periodic lateralized epileptiform discharges on EEG. Atrophic change of wide sylvian fissure, and low attenuation area over right frontal and temporal lobes are detected on CT (**a**). Proton density MR image shows high intensity signal area around the right sylvian fissure and insular cortex (**b**).

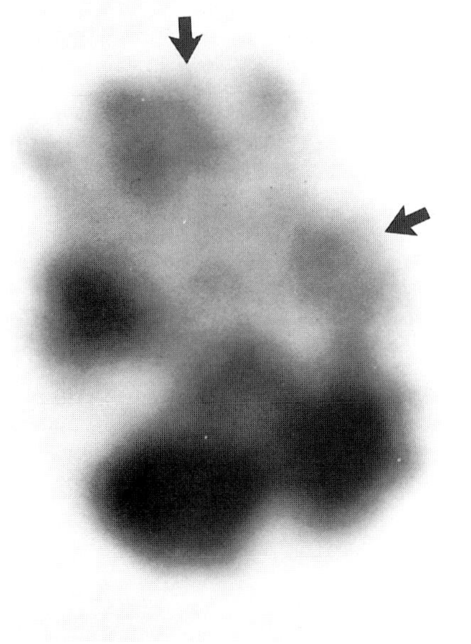

Fig. 8. Rasmussen syndrome. An 8-year-old boy with epilepsia partialis continua and complex partial seizures underwent temporal lobectomy from which Rasmussen syndrome was pathologically diagnosed. Interictal SPECT shows diffuse decreased rCBF over the left frontal and temporal regions (arrows).

pediatric patients [67]. MRI demonstrated increased intensity signal in a right insula and atrophic change around the ipsilateral sylvian fissure in a recent patient with epilepsia partialis continua, progressive left hemiparesis and periodic lateralized epileptiform discharges on EEG. CT scan shows only atrophic changes localized to the temporal region (fig. 7). SPECT showed decreased rCBF over right frontotemporal lobes (fig. 8).

Two patients with the Rasmussen syndrome were examined with MRI in a recent review [83]. Proton density MRI demonstrated focally localized increased intensity signals in the white matter, associated with hemiatrophy. MRI was better able to evaluate the extent of the disease and the evolution of the disorder. In 6 patients studied with PET and SPECT, the characteristic findings were a regional decrease in glucose metabolism with a focal increase in LCMRglc on PET, and a regional decrease in rCBF with a focal increase correlating with the epileptogenic area on SPECT [37].

Infantile Spasms (West Syndrome)

The West syndrome consists of infantile spasms, arrest of psychomotor development and hypsarrhythmia, and is proposed as generalized cryptogenic or symptomatic epilepsies and epileptic syndrome (age-related) [18]. The spasms may be characterized by flexor, extensor, or mixed flexion-extension jerks, lightning, or nods. Onset peaks between 4 and 7 months of life, and always occurs before the age of 1 year.

In this institute in a retrospective review of the last 4 years (1987–1991), there were 49 patients with a clinical and electrophysiological diagnosis of infantile spasms. CT had abnormal findings in 13 out of 20 patients, consisting of a diffuse atrophic change in 6 and a focal change in 7. Five of 9 patients examined with MRI had focal abnormalities consisting of pachygyria. Twenty patients were interictally studied with SPECT, demonstrating focal decreased rCBF in 2 and increased rCBF in 5, multifocal decrease in 8, diffuse decrease in 3, and the remaining 3 showed normal SPECT. Of the 3 patients who had immediate postictal SPECT, all 3 showed focal increased rCBF corresponding to the epileptogenic area on EEG (fig. 9).

The metabolic function study of PET has been reported being useful in order to resolve the spatial focus coincidence to EEG focus. PET with FDG could identify the abnormality of local cerebral glucose metabolism in 5

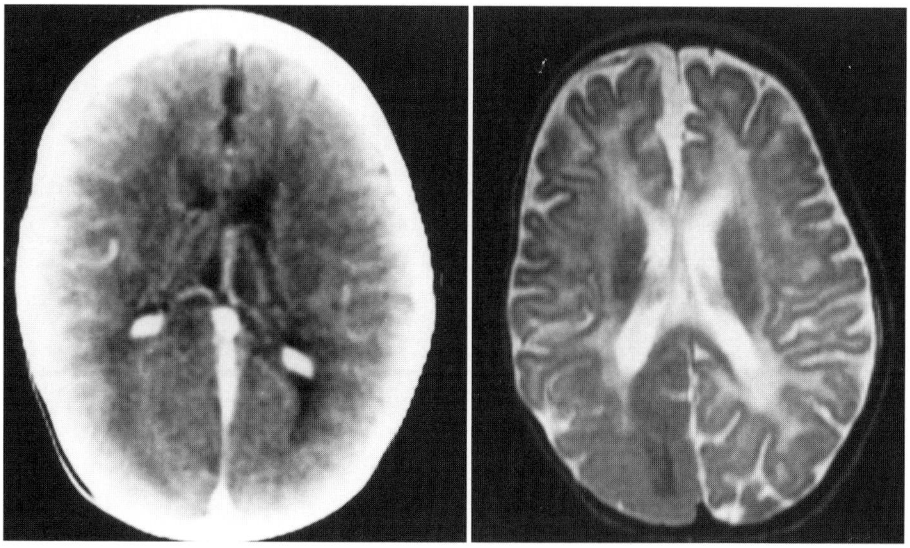

Fig. 9. Infantile spasms, focal cortical dysplasia. A 7-month-old girl with infantile spasms and left partial motor seizures followed by Todd's palsy; EEG showed electrodecremental events as well as hemispheric modified hypsarrhythmia over right hemisphere. CT shows asymmetrical posterior lateral ventricle, with unremarkable changes of cortex (**a**). T_2W MRI shows pachygyria and loss of gray and white matter differentiation over right occipital and posterior temporal regions (**b**).

out of 13 children with cryptogenic infantile spasms; the cortical hypometabolism on PET corresponding to the epileptogenic focus allows one to proceed to surgical excision under electrocorticography [15].

Discussion

Computed Tomography

CT is superior in revealing calcified structural lesions including benign temporal neoplasms, and less successful in demonstrating MTS or congenital abnormalities. The long-standing neoplasms in temporal lobe producing intractable complex partial seizures include low grade astrocytoma, ganglioglioma, oligodendroglioma, and rarely mixed glioma. They enhance poorly with intravenous contrast, and the small calcifications are better demonstrated on thin slice coronal CT [62]. In the patients with the Sturge-Weber syndrome, gyriform calcification which corresponds to epileptogenic focus could be seen on CT in infancy [59, 90]. However, the other type of congenital abnormalities such as neuronal migration disorders (pachygyria and agyria, lissencephaly) were difficult to detect on CT. Major findings of calcifications of tuberous sclerosis do not always correspond to the seizure focus. In the ptients with MTS and Rasmussen syndrome, CT cannot detect abnormal findings in localized epileptogenic regions.

Xenon CT

Xenon CT demonstrates blood flow to different regions of the brain similar to SPECT. However, xenon CT has the advantage that anatomical CT slices are compared to the localization of abnormal perfusion in the patients with seizure disorders [87, 89]. In addition, blood flow can be exactly measured on the basis of xenon concentration, which cannot be done with SPECT [35, 42, 95]. The disadvantages of xenon CT are the discomfort of patients who also have to be cooperative and the limited number of scans that can be performed in each study.

Magnetic Resonance Imaging

Neuronal migration disorders representing cortical heterotopia, agyria, pachygyria and schizencephaly are detected on MRI, which is an excellent tool for diagnosing the abnormal cortex and underlying gray-white matter interface [61]. The presence of macroscopic heterotopic gray matter is well known to be frequently associated with seizure disorders in pediatric patients [77]. Specificity and sensitivity of MRI in terms of cortical dysplasia in temporal lobe epilepsy were reported as being high, and MRI could detect abnormal neuronal migration, most of which produced epileptogenic foci [46]. MRI is considered to be the best imaging method in the investigation of the pediatric patient with congenital abnormalities.

MTS is the most common pathological abnormality encountered in temporal lobectomy in the patients with intractable complex partial seizure [33]. Reports varied about the mesial temporal gliosis and the prevalence of abnormal increased intensity signal changes on T2-weighted MR images. T2 abnormalities were reported in 11 of 14 patients with MTS, and in 6 of 12 patients with mild to moderate gliosis of the hippocampus [45]. On the other hand, no abnormalities were found on MRI in 18 patients with mesial temporal gliosis reported by Sperling et al. [78]; Brooks et al. [13] also reported the insensitivity of MRI in MTS in patients with complex partial seizures, namely that 35 of 38 patients with mesial temporal gliosis had no signal abnormalities. Coronal views on MRI are the most useful views to reveal the details of the mesial temporal region without the bony artifacts seen on CT. This is an essential technique to evaluate pathological changes in the hippocampus. In patients with refractory temporal lobe epilepsy, there is asymmetry in the size of the temporal lobes which can be measured, the smaller temporal lobes correlating with the seizure focus, particularly with a unilateral focus [55], whereas other authors had standardized volumetric MRI data demonstrating differences of hippocampal volumes correlating with the side of the focus [40, 41].

Single Photon Emission Computed Tomography

SPECT findings correlate favorably with localization-related epilepsy on EEG, demonstrating the interictal hypoperfusion corresponding to the immediate postictal hyperperfusion. The analysis of interictal and postictal SPECT using ^{99m}Tc HMPAO recordings can therefore improve to focusing epileptogenic areas, especially in the patients without any structural lesions [73, 79]. This is where SPECT imaging is most important and useful. The SPECT scan shows rCBF changes contributing to functional localization of the epileptogenic focus. Even when CT and MRI show no abnormality in infancy and childhood with localized epiletogenic focus at the early stage, interictal and postictal change of rCBF on SPECT with ^{99m}Tc HMPAO may demonstrate corresponding epileptogenic focus on EEG.

Positron Emission Tomography

The LCMRglc can be measured with PET. In the patients with refractory seizures, PET showed a hypometabolic zone larger than the lesions found on MRI [85]. Structural lesions in temporal lobes, the majority of which were MTS, area of involvement by other imaging modalities were smaller than the area of hypometabolism seen on PET [8, 23]. The abnormal findings of structural lesions on MRI and CT have not been proved to be an epileptogenic focus, because epilepsy is a disease of altered function, not structure [85]. PET has been reported to effectively detect the epileptogenic area. Chugani [15] dramatically highlighted abnormal hypometabolism on parietooccipital-temporal region in 5 infants with cryptogenic infantile spasm, followed by resective surgery offering improved prognosis.

Radiopharmaceutical Studies

Neurotransmitter and receptor disorders have been investigated with radiolabeled ligands on SPECT or PET in experimental models of neuropharmacology and neurobiology [54]. The benzodiazepine-inverse agonist, iodine-123-labeled Ro 16-0154, enables SPECT investigations of central benzodiazepine receptors in human brain [7, 38]. A reduction in the cortical benzodiazepine receptor density in the epileptogenic foci of patients with partial seizures was demonstrated, whereas a focal alteration of cortical inhibition was not a prominent feature of the patients with generalized seizures [75]. Although these frontiers will have to be studied further for clinical epilepsy, initially benzodiazepine mapping with SPECT seems to be helpful in order to identify localization-related epilepsy [5].

Combination of Neuroimaging and Electrophysiological Study

With advances in three-dimensional (3-D) neuroimaging, functional anatomy has been demonstrated experimentally [16]. It is possible to visualize significant functional metabolic changes in a naturalistic 3-D format, by computer-based image analysis. Currently determination of international ten-twenty system electrode locations on MRI with markers provides analyses of electrodes which correspond to epileptiform activities, to aid localization of epileptogenic focus [47]. In the future 3-D neuroimaging will produce correlations of structural anatomy, functional and electrophysiological, furthermore the density of neurotransmitters and the biochemical reactions may be added in order to identify a focus of the epilepsy.

Magnetoencephalogram

In children with intractable seizures, there is interest in noninvasive localization methods which are accurate and sensitive to localize the focus of seizure onset. The magnetoencephalogram (MEG) has been developed for physical interpretation of fields by dipole localization, the mapping of which can resolve the center of active currents. The localization and detection of the epileptic focus may be improved by the MEG, because (1) localization in MEG is generally simpler than in EEG, (2) MEG and EEG each are more sensitive to different orientations of intracranial currents, and (3) the combination of MEG and EEG can increase the certainty of localization [19, 82, 93].

Proposal

The pediatric patient with intractable seizures should be monitored with EEG and more special EEG to detect focal epileptiform activity interictally and postictally. Localization-related epilepsy is confirmed with MRI first for the anatomical study of structural lesions. If MRI does not have any abnormal findings, CT should be performed for possible missed calcified lesions. Physiological study, SPECT, PET, Xe CT are helpful to identify the interictal hypometabolism over the epileptogenic area, in addition to the interictal and postictal SPECT, even if structural lesions are not found. 3-D imaging combined with subdural, even conventional scalp EEG and neuroimaging as well as MEG are helpful for the mapping of epileptogenic areas for epilepsy surgery.

References

1 Aguilar MJ, Rasmussen T: Role of encephalitis in pathogenesis of epilepsy. AMA Arch Neurol 1960;2:663–676.
2 Ashtari M, Barr WB, Schaul N, et al: Three-dimensional fast low-angle shot imaging and computerized volume measurement of the hippocampus in patients with chronic epilepsy of the temporal lobe. AJNR 1991;12:941–947.
3 Babb TL, Brown WJ: Pathological findings in epilepsy; in Engel J Jr (ed): Surgical Treatment of the Epilepsies. New York, Raven Press, 1987, pp 511–540.
4 Barkovich AJ, Chuang SH, Norman D: MR of neuronal migration abnormalies. AJNR 1987; 8:1009–1017.
5 Bartenstein P, Ludolph A, Schober O, et al: Benzodiazepine receptors and cerebral blood flow in partial epilepsy. Eur J Nucl Med 1991; 18:111–118.
6 Barth PG: Disorders of cerebral migration. Can J Neurol Sci 1987;14:1–16.
7 Beer HF, Blauenstein PA, Hasler PH, et al: In vitro and in vivo evaluation of iodine-123-Ro 16-0154: A new imaging agent for SPECT investigations of benzodiazepine receptors. J Nucl Med 1990;31:1007–1014.
8 Bernardi S, Trimble MR, Frackowiak RSJ, et al: An interictal study of partial epilepsy using positron emission tomography and the oxygen-15 inhalation technique. J Neurol Neurosurg Psychiatry 1983;46:473–477.
9 Bignami A, Palladini G, Zappella M: Unilateral megarencephaly with nerve cell hypertrophy. An anatomical and quantitative histochemical study. Brain Res 1969;9:103–114.
10 Bourneville DM: Sclérose tubéreuse des circonvolutions cérébrales: Idiotie et épilepsie hémiplégique. Arch Neurol (Paris) 1880;1:81091.
11 Brewis M, Poskanzer D, Rolland C, et al: Neurological disease in an English city. Acta Neurol Scand 1966;42(suppl 24):1–89.
12 Bronen RA, Cheung G, Charles JT, et al: Imaging findings in hippocampal sclerosis: Correlation with pathology. AJNR 1991;12:933–940.
13 Brooks BS, King DW, Gammel TEL, et al: MR imaging in patients with intractable complex partial epileptic seizures. AJNR 1990;11:93–99.
14 Cavanaugh JB, Meyer A: Aetiological aspects of Ammon's horn sclerosis associated with temporal lobe epilepsy. Br Med J 1956;ii: 1403.
15 Chugani HT, Shields WD, Shewmon DA, et al: Infantile spasm. 1. PET identifies focal cortical dysgenesis in cryptogenic cases for surgical treatment. Ann Neurol 1990;27:406–413.
16 Collins RC, Santori EM, Toga AW: A three-dimensional image of brain function; in Toga AW (ed): Three-Dimensional Neuroimaging. New York, Raven Press, 1990, pp 149–164.
17 Commission on Classification and Terminology of the International Leage against Epilepsy: Proposal for classification of epilepsies. Epilepsia 1981;26/3:268–278.
18 Commission on Classification and Terminology of the International Leage against Epilepsy: Proposal for revised classification of epilepsies and epileptic syndromes. Epilepsia 1989;30: 389–399.
19 Cuffin BN, Cohen D: Comparison and treatment of intractable seizures. Cleve Clin Q 1984;2:227–240.
20 Dambska M, Wisniewski K, Sher JH: An autopsy case of hemimegalencephaly. Brain Dev 1984;6:60–64.
21 Dorne HL, O'Gorman AM, Melanson D: Computed tomography of intracranial gangliogliomas. AJNR 1986;7:281–285.
22 Drake J, Hoffman HJ, Kobayashi J, et al: Surgical management of children with temporal lobe epilepsy and mass lesions. Neurosurgery 1987;21:792–797.
23 Engel J Jr, Brown WJ, Kuhl DE, et al: Pathological findings underlying focal temporal lobe hypometabolism in partial epilepsy. Ann Neurol 1982;12:518–529.
24 Falconer MA, Taylor DC: Surgical treatment of drug resistant epilepsy due to medial temporal sclerosis. Arch Neurol 1968;19:353–361.
25 Fitz CR, Harwood-Nash DC, Boldt DW: The radiographic features of unilateral megarencephaly. Neuroradiology 1978;15:145–148.
26 Fitz CC: Tuberous sclerosis; in Hoffman HJ (ed): Disorders of the Developing Nervous System: Diagnosis and Treatment. Boston, Blackwell, 1986; pp 607–616.
27 Friede RL: Dysplasias of cerebral cortex; in Friede RL (ed): Developmental neuropathology. Wien, Springer, 1975, pp 297–313.
28 Gammel TE, Adams RJ: Modified CT techniques in the evaluation of temporal lobe epilepsy prior to lobectomy. AJNR 1987;8:131–134.
29 Garrido E, Becker LE, Hoffman HJ, et al: Gangliogliomas in children: A clinicopathological study. Childs Brain 1978;4:339–346.
30 Gastaut H: So called 'psychomotor' and 'temporal' epilepsy. Epilepsia 1953;2:59–99.
31 Gates JR, Cruz-Rodriguez R: Mesial temporal sclerosis: Pathogenesis, diagnosis, and management. Epilepsia 1990;31(suppl 3);S55–S66.
32 George RE, Hoffman HJ, Hwang PA, et al: Management of intractable seizures in unilateral megarencephaly. J Epilepsy 1990;3(Suppl): 305–313.
33 Glaser GH: Treatment of intractable temporal lobe-limbic epilepsy (complex partial seizures) by temporal lobectomy. Ann Neurol 1980;46: 964–970.
34 Gupta PC, Roy S, Tandon PN: Progressive epilepsy due to chronic persistent encephalitis. Report of four cases. J Neurol Sci 1974;22: 105–120.
35 Gur D, Yonas H, Good WF: Local cerebral blood flow by xenon-enhanced CT: Current status, potential improvements, and future directions. Cerebrovasc Brain Metab Rev 1989; 1:68–86.
36 Hwang PA, Gilday DL, Adams C, et al: SPECT studies in epilepsy: Application to epilepsy surgery in children. J Epilepsy, (in press).
37 Hwang PA, Gilday DL, Spire J-P, et al: Chronic focal encephalitis of Rasmussen: Functional neuroimaging studies with positron emission tomography and single-photon emission computed tomography scanning; in Anderman F (ed): Chronic Focal Encephalitis and Epilepsy: Rasmussen's Syndrome. Boston, Butterworth-Heinemann, 1991, pp 61–72.
38 Innis RB, Al-Tikriti MS, Zoghbi SS, et al: SPECT imaging of the benzodiazepine receptor: Feasibility of in vivo potency measurements from stepwise displacement curves (see comments). J Nucl Med 1991;32:1762–1763.
39 Jabbari R, Gundersib CH, Wippold F, et al: Magnetic resonance imaging in partial complex epilepsy. Arch Neurol 1986;43:869–872.
40 Jack CR, Sharbrough FW, Twomey CK, et al: Temporal lobe seizures: Lateralization with MR volume measurements of the hippocampal formation. Radiology 1990;175:423–429.
41 Jack CR, Sharbrough FW, Cascino GD, et al: Magnetic resonance image-based hippocampal volumetry: Correlation with outcome after temporal lobectomy. Ann Neurol 1992;31: 138–146.
42 Johnson DW, Stringer WA, Marks MP, et al: Stable xenon CT cerebral blood flow imaging: Rationale for and role in clinical decision making. AJNR 1991;12:201–213.

43 Kalifa GL, Chiron C, Sellier N, et al: Hemimegalencephaly: MR imaging in five children. Radiology 1987;165:29–33.
44 King M, Stephenson JBP, Ziervogel M, et al: Hemimegalencephaly – A case for hemispherectomy? Neuropediatrics 1985;16:46–55.
45 Kuzniecky R, Sayette V, Ethier R, et al: Magnetic resonance imaging in temporal lobe epilepsy: Pathological correlations. Ann Neurol 1987;22:341–347.
46 Kuzniecky R, Garcia JH, Faught E, et al: Cortical dysplasia in temporal lobe epilepsy: Magnetic resonance imaging correlations. Ann Neurol 1991;29:293–298.
47 Lagerlund TD, Sharbrough FW, Jack CR, et al: Determination of 10–20 system electrode locations using MRI scanning with markers (abstract). American Electroencephalographic Society, 1991, p 119.
48 Latack JT, Abou-Khalil BW, Siegel GJ, et al: Patients with partial seizures: Evaluation by MR, CT, and PET imaging. Radiology 1986; 159:159–163.
49 Laurence KM: A case of unilateral megarencephaly. Dev Med Child Neurol 1964;6:585–590.
50 Lévesque MF, Nakasato N, Vinters HV, et al: Surgical treatment of limbic epilepsy associated with extrahippocampal lesions: The problem of dual pathology. J Neurosurg 1991;75: 364–370.
51 Lund M: On epilepsy in Sturge-Weber's disease. Acta Psychiatr Neurol 1949;24:578–586.
52 Manz HJ, Phillips TM, Rowden G, et al: Unilateral megalencephaly, cerebral cortical dysplasia, neuronal hypertrophy, and heterotopia: Cytomorphometric, fluorometric cytochemical, and biochemical analyses. Acta Neuropathol (Berl) 1979;45:97–103.
53 Margerison JH, Corsellis JAN: Epilepsy and the temporal lobe epilepsy. Brain 1966;89: 499–530.
54 Maziere B, Maziere M: Where have we got to with neuroreceptor mapping of the human brain? Eur J Nucl Med 1990;16:817–835.
55 McLachlan RS, Nicholson RL, Black S, et al: Nuclear magnetic resonance imaging, a new approach to the investigation of refractory temporal lobe epilepsy. Epilepsia 1985;26:555–562.
56 Meyer FB, Marsh WR, Laws ER, et al: Temporal lobectomy in children with epilepsy. J Neurosurg 1986;64:371–376.
57 Mikhael MA, Mattar AG: Malformation of the cerebral cortex with heterotopia of the gray matter. J Comput Assist Tomogr 1978;2:291–296.
58 Nixon JR, Houser OW, Gomez MR, et al: Cerebral tuberous sclerosis: MR imaging. Radiology 1989;170:869–873.
59 Ogunmekan AO, Hwang PA, Hoffman HJ: Sturge-Weber-Dimitri disease: Role of hemispherectomy in prognosis. Can J Neurol Sci 1989;16:78–80.
60 Ormson MJ, Kispert DB, Sharbrough FW, et al: Cryptic structural lesions in refractory partial epilepsy: MR imaging and CT studies. Radiology 1986;160:215–219.
61 Osborn RE, Byrd SE, Naidich TP, et al: MR imaging of neuronal migration disorders. AJNR 1988;9:1101–1106.
62 Otsubo H, Hoffman HJ, Humphreys RP, et al: Evaluation, surgical approach and outcome of seizure patients with ganglioglioma. Pediatr Neurosurg 1990–1991;16:208–212.
63 Oxbury JM, Adams CBT: Neurosurgery for epilepsy. Br J Hosp Med 1989;41:372–377.
64 Palmini A, Anderman F, Olivier A, et al: Focal neuronal migration disorders and intractable partial epilepsy: A study of 30 patients. Ann Neurol 1991;30:741–749.
65 Palmini A, Anderman F, Olivier A, et al: Focal neuronal migration disorders and intractable partial epilepsy: Results of surgical treatment. Ann Neurol 1991;30:750–757.
66 Penfield W, Jasper H: Epilepsy and the Functional Anatomy of the Human Brain. Boston Little, Brown, 1954.
67 Piatt JH, Hwang PA, Armstrong DC, et al: Chronic focal encephalitis (Rasmussen syndrome): Six cases. Epilepsia 1988;29:268–279.
68 Rasmussen T, Olszewski J, Loyd-Smith D: Focal seizures due to chronic localized encephalitis. Neurology 1968;8:435–445.
69 Rasmussen T, McCann W: Clinical studies of patients with focal epilepsy due to 'chronic encephalitis'. Trans Am Neurol Assoc 1968;93: 89–94.
70 Rasmussen T: Surgery of epilepsy associated with brain tumors. Adv Neurol 1975;8:227–239.
71 Robain O, Floquet CH, Heldt N, et al: Hemimegalencephaly: A clinicopathological study of four cases. Neuropathol Appl Neurobiol 1988; 14:125–135.
72 Rochkind S, Hoffman HJ, Hendrick EB: Sturge-Weber syndrome: Natural history and prognosis. J Epilepsy 1990;3(suppl):293–304.
73 Rowe CC, Berkovic SF, Sia STB, et al: Localization epileptic foci with postictal single photon emission computed tomography. Ann Neurol 1989;26:660–668.
74 Sano K, Malamud N: Clinical significance of sclerosis of the cornu ammonis. Arch Neurol Psychiatry 1953;70:40–53.
75 Savic I, Widen L, Thorell JO, et al: Cortical benzodiazepine receptor binding in patients with generalized and partial epilepsy. Epilepsia 1990;31:724–730.
76 Schörner W, Meencke H-J, Felix R: Temporal lobe epilepsy: Comparison of CT and MR imaging. AJNR 1987;149:1231–1239.
77 Smith AS, Weinstein MA, Quencer RM, et al: Association of heterotopic gray matter with seizures: MR imaging. Radiology 1988;168:195–198.
78 Sperling MR, Wilson G, Engel J Jr, et al: Magnetic resonance imaging in intractable partial epilepsy: Correlative studies. Ann Neurol 1986;20:57–62.
79 Stefan H, Pawlik G, Bócher-Schwarz HG, et al: Functional and morphological abnormalities in temporal lobe epilepsy: A comparison of interictal and ictal EEG, CT, MRI, SPECT and PET. J Neurol 1987;234:377–384.
80 Stefan H, Bauer J, Feistel H, et al: Regional cerebral blood flow during focal seizures of temporal and frontocentral onset. Ann Neurol 1990;27:406–413.
81 Sturge W: A case of partial epilepsy, apparently due to a lesion of one of the vasomotor centers of the brain. Trans Clin Soc Lond 1879;12: 162–167.
82 Sutherling WW, Barth DS: Magnetoencephalography in clinical epilepsy studies UCLA experience; in Sato S (ed): Advances in Neurology. 54. Magnetoencephalography. New York, Raven Press, 1990; pp 231–245.
83 Tampieri D, Melanson D, Ethier R: Imaging of chronic encephalitis; in Anderman F (ed): Chronic Focal Encephalitis and Epilepsy: Rasmussen's Syndrome. Boston, Butterworth-Heineman, 1991, pp 47–60.
84 Taylor D, Falconer M, Burton C, et al: Focal cortical dysplasia of the cerebral cortex in epilepsy. J Neurol Neurosurg Psychiatry 1971;34: 369–387.
85 Theodore WH, Dorwart R, Holmes M, et al: Neuroimaging in refractory partial seizures: Comparison of PET, CT, and MRI. Neurology 1986;36:750–759.
86 Tjiam AT, Stefanko S, Schenk VWD, et al: Infantile spasms associated with hemihypsarrhythmia and hemimegalencephaly. Dev Med Child Neurol 1978;20:779–798.
87 Touho H, Karasawa J, Shishido H, et al: Stable xenon CT-CBF study with measurement of end-tidal xenon concentration – Correlation by arterial concentration of xenon. No To Shinkei 1989;41:603–609.
88 Townsend JJ, Nielsen SL, Malamud N: Unilateral megarencephaly: Hamartoma or neoplasm? Neurology 1975;25:448–453.
89 Uchida K, Tamura K, Takayama H, et al: Xenon-enhanced CT CBF measurement in intracranial vascular malformations. No Shinkei Geka 1989;17:239–246.
90 Venes JL: Sturge-Weber syndrome, in Hoffman HJ, Epstein F (eds): Disorders of the Developing Nervous System: Diagnosis and Treatment. Boston, Blackwell, 1986, pp 617–623.
91 Voght H: Zur Diagnostik der tuberosen Sklerose. Z Erforsch Behandl Jugendl Schwachsinns 1908;2:1–12.
92 Weber FP: Right sided hemi-hypertrophy resulting from right-sided congenital spastic hemiplegia, with morbid condition of the left side of the brain revealed by radiograms. J Neurol Psychopathol 1922;3:134–139.
93 Wood CC, Cohen D, Cuffin BN, et al: Electrical sources in the human somatosensory cortex: Identification by combined magnetic and electrical potential recordings. Science 1985; 227:1051–1053.
94 Wyler AR, Bolender N: Preoperative CT diagnosis of mesial temporal sclerosis for surgical treatment of epilepsy. Ann Neurol 1983;13:59–64.
95 Yonas H, Darby JM, Marks EC, et al: CBF measured by Xe-CT: Approach to analysis and normal values. J Cereb Blood Flow Metab 1991;11:716–725.

Concepts in Pediatric Neurosurgery (ISSN 0251–2068)
Edited by the American Society for Pediatric Neurosurgery

Editor:
Arthur E. Marlin

Concepts in Pediatric Neurosurgery 11

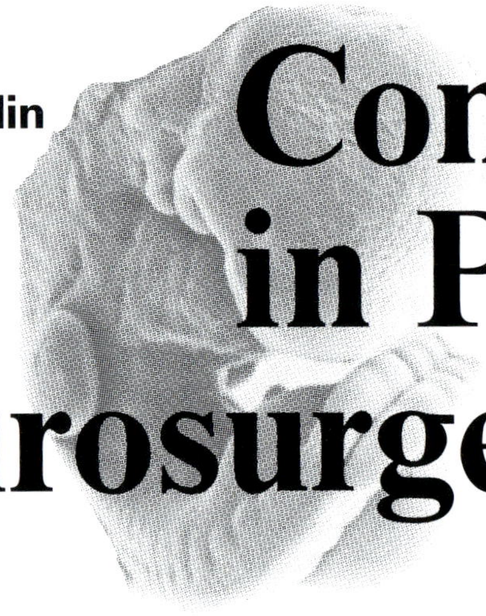

This stimulating and well-illustrated volume features 15 papers presented by leading neurosurgeons at the 1990 annual meeting of the American Society for Pediatric Neurosurgery. The authors discuss the latest concepts and exchange valuable clinical experiences on diverse neurological disorders affecting children. Controversial questions of diagnosis and management are addressed and results with new surgical and imaging procedures are reported. Topics covered include cervical dysraphic abnormalities, CSF shunts and shunt infections, pediatric brain tumors as well as stereotaxic balloon encephalotomy and gadolinium-enhanced magnetic resonance imaging of brain tumor patients.
Contributing to a better understanding of pediatric neurosurgical problems, the opinions, ideas and innovations contained in this book offer neurosurgeons, neurologists and pediatricians competent and thought-provoking reading.

Contents

Fields of Interest
Neurology, Neurosurgery; Pediatrics; Oncology, Pathology, Surgery

Concepts in Pediatric Neurosurgery 11
Editor: Marlin, A.E. (San Antonio, Tex.)
VIII + 166 p., 63 fig., 23 tab., hard cover, 1991
SFr. 215.– / DM 257.– / £ 93.50 / US$ 172.00
US$ price for USA, £ price for UK only (subject to change)
ISBN 3–8055–5328–5

KARGER